Teen Health Series

Skin Health Information for Teens, Third Edition

Skin Health Information for Teens, Third Edition

Health Tips About Dermatological Disorders And Activities
That Affect the Skin, Hair, And Nails

Including Facts About Acne, Infectious Skin Conditions, Skin Cancer,
Skin Injuries, And Other Conditions And Lifestyle Choices, Such as
Tanning, Tattooing, and Piercing

Edited by Lisa Esposito

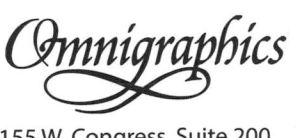

155 W. Congress, Suite 200
Detroit, MI 48226

Bibliographic Note

Because this page cannot legibly accommodate all the copyright notices, the Bibliographic Note portion of the Preface constitutes an extension of the copyright notice.

Edited by Lisa Esposito

Teen Health Series

Karen Bellenir, *Managing Editor*
David A. Cooke, M.D., *Medical Consultant*
Elizabeth Collins, *Research and Permissions Coordinator*
EdIndex, *Services for Publishers, Indexers*

* * *

Omnigraphics, Inc.

Matthew P. Barbour, *Senior Vice President*
Kevin M. Hayes, *Operations Manager*

* * *

Peter E. Ruffner, *Publisher*

Copyright © 2013 Omnigraphics, Inc.
ISBN 978-0-7808-1317-5
E-ISBN 978-0-7808-1318-2

Library of Congress Cataloging-in-Publication Data

Skin health information for teens : health tips about dermatological disorders and activities that affect the skin, hair, and nails : including facts about acne, infectious skin conditions, skin cancer, skin injuries, and other conditions and lifestyle choices, such as tanning, tattooing, and piercing / edited by Lisa Esposito. -- Third edition.
     pages cm. -- (Teen health series)
  Audience: Grade 9 to 12.
  Summary: "Provides basic consumer health information for teens about acne, infections, and other skin conditions, with facts about skin cancer prevention and tips for taking care of the skin, nails, and hair. Includes index, resource information, and recommendations for further reading"-- Provided by publisher.
  Includes bibliographical references and index.
  ISBN 978-0-7808-1317-5 (hardcover : alk. paper) 1. Teenagers--Health and hygiene. 2. Skin--Care and hygiene. 3. Beauty, Personal. I. Esposito, Lisa, editor.
  RA777.S546 2013
  616.5'00835--dc23
                                                                                          2013009908

Table of Contents

Part Four: Other Diseases And Disorders Affecting The Skin

Part Five: Skin Injuries

Part Six: Taking Care Of Your Skin, Hair, And Nails

Part Seven: If You Need More Information

Preface

About This Book

From the thinnest layer of skin on the eyelids to the thickest layer on the soles of the feet, skin protects the entire body and is essential to survival. But skin itself is vulnerable to rashes, infections, injuries, and disease, from the relatively minor to the extremely serious. Coping with diseases like skin cancer and scleroderma can leave teens overwhelmed and desperate for information. And while conditions like acne and vitiligo are not physically threatening, they can be emotionally devastating at a period when appearance is all-important. Other conditions that might seem harmless—like birthmarks, blushing, and excess sweating—also can affect self-esteem. In addition, teens make choices about sun and outdoor exposure, body art, and beauty products that have the potential to damage the skin's health and weaken its protective ability.

Skin Health Information For Teens, Third Edition provides updated information on medical conditions that affect the skin, hair, and nails. It describes the basics of healthy skin and skin care, taking different skin types into account. It explains prevention, warning signs, and treatment options for skin cancer and spells out the risks of tanning—outside and indoors. Acne is discussed in depth, including scar treatment and developing a healthy self-image even with facial skin that is "different." Care of common conditions—such as allergic rashes, viral infections like cold sores, and injuries like cuts, scrapes, bruises, bites, and stings—is also covered. Information to help teens make healthy choices as they express themselves through cosmetics, piercing, and tattoos is also included. Finally, the book provides a section on further reading about skin concerns and a directory of additional resources.

How To Use This Book

This book is divided into parts and chapters. Parts focus on broad areas of interest; chapters are devoted to single topics within a part.

Part One: Skin Basics provides information about skin anatomy and the skin's protective function. It discusses why freckles and brown spots occur and how teens blush. It includes information on ethnicity and specific skin conditions. Appearance concerns and healthy body image for teens with facial differences—such as birthmarks and scars—are addressed, and the effects of smoking on looks are described.

Part Two: Acne focuses on the causes of acne and how it develops in teens. It details treatments such as over-the-counter products, prescription medicines, and dermatologic procedures for treating acne scars. Gender-specific tips on coping with acne are provided, and the psychological effects of acne are discussed.

Part Three: Infectious Conditions Of The Skin describes bacterial, viral, fungal, and parasitic diseases that affect the skin. Bacterial concerns include impetigo and necrotizing fasciitis, the so-called flesh-eating disease. The viral conditions addressed include cold sores, warts, and human papillomavirus (HPV). Chapters related to fungal and parasitic infections discuss ringworm, athlete's foot, Lyme disease, scabies, and others.

Part Four: Other Disorders And Diseases Affecting The Skin discusses a variety of inherited, allergic, autoimmune, and other skin disorders. It explains conditions that are medically benign but cause for concern in self-conscious teens, such as cellulite, stretch marks, vitiligo, rosacea, and hyperhidrosis (excessive sweating). It also describes itching, hives, eczema, lupus, scleroderma, psoriasis, and moles. Skin cancer—particularly melanoma and basal cell carcinoma—is detailed, including causes, detection, diagnosis, treatment, and prevention.

Part Five: Skin Injuries provides facts about prevention, first aid, and treatment of scrapes, cuts, bruises, insect bites and stings, animal bites, poison ivy and poison oak, and frostbite. It covers care of stitches, scars and scar removal, corns and calluses, and nail abnormalities. Burn assessment and treatment are explained, along with a section on prevention of burn injuries in teen workers. Skin picking is described and coping mechanisms are suggested.

Part Six: Taking Care Of Your Skin, Hair, And Nails describes self-care and lifestyle choices teens make that affect their appearance and health. It details concerns about outdoor and indoor tanning and offers facts about tanning alternatives. Safety precautions are given for teens interested in tattoos or piercing. Hair health, including damage from flat irons and hair-care products, and hair loss are discussed. Nail care and abnormalities are also addressed.

Part Seven: If You Need More Information provides suggestions for additional reading on topics related to skin and a list of further resources.

Bibliographic Note

This volume contains documents and excerpts from publications issued by the following government agencies: Centers for Disease Control and Prevention (CDC); National Cancer Institute; National Institute of Arthritis and Musculoskeletal and Skin Diseases; National Library of Medicine; Occupational Health and Safety Administration; Office on Women's

Health; Substance Abuse And Mental Health Services Administration (SAMHSA); and the U.S. Food and Drug Administration (FDA).

In addition, this volume contains copyrighted documents and articles produced by the following organizations: Action on Smoking and Health (ASH): A.D.A.M., Inc.; Akron Children's Hospital; American Academy of Dermatology; American College of Rheumatology; American Osteopathic College of Dermatology; American Society of Health-System Pharmacists; Boston Children's Hospital Center for Young Women's Health; Canadian Paediatric Society; Cleveland Clinic; Columbia St. Mary's Regional Burn Center; Louisiana State University School of Veterinary Medicine; National Health Service, U.K Department of Health; National Psoriasis Foundation; Nemours Foundation; New Zealand Dermatological Society; Palo Alto Medical Foundation; PEW Center on the States; Trichotillomania Learning Center; Vivacare; Vitiligo Support International; Women's and Children's Health Network, Government of South Australia; and the Women's Dermatologic Society.

The photograph on the front cover is © iStockphoto via Thinkstock.

Full citation information is provided on the first page of each chapter. Every effort has been made to secure all necessary rights to reprint the copyrighted material. If any omissions have been made, please contact Omnigraphics to make corrections for future editions.

Acknowledgements

In addition to the organizations listed above, special thanks are due to Liz Collins, research and permissions coordinator; Karen Bellenir, managing editor; and WhimsyInk, prepress services provider.

About The *Teen Health Series*

At the request of librarians serving today's young adults, the *Teen Health Series* was developed as a specially focused set of volumes within Omnigraphics' *Health Reference Series*. Each volume deals comprehensively with a topic selected according to the needs and interests of people in middle school and high school.

Teens seeking preventive guidance, information about disease warning signs, medical statistics, and risk factors for health problems will find answers to their questions in the *Teen Health Series*. The *Series*, however, is not intended to serve as a tool for diagnosing illness, in prescribing treatments, or as a substitute for the physician/patient relationship. All people concerned about medical symptoms or the possibility of disease are encouraged to seek professional care from an appropriate health care provider.

If there is a topic you would like to see addressed in a future volume of the *Teen Health Series*, please write to:

Editor
Teen Health Series
Omnigraphics, Inc.
155 W. Congress, Suite 200
Detroit, MI 48226

A Note About Spelling And Style

Teen Health Series editors use *Stedman's Medical Dictionary* as an authority for questions related to the spelling of medical terms and the *Chicago Manual of Style* for questions related to grammatical structures, punctuation, and other editorial concerns. Consistent adherence is not always possible, however, because the individual volumes within the *Series* include many documents from a wide variety of different producers and copyright holders, and the editor's primary goal is to present material from each source as accurately as is possible following the terms specified by each document's producer. This sometimes means that information in different chapters or sections may follow other guidelines and alternate spelling authorities. For example, occasionally a copyright holder may require that eponymous terms be shown in possessive forms (Crohn's disease *vs.* Crohn disease) or that British spelling norms be retained (leukaemia *vs.* leukemia).

Locating Information Within The *Teen Health Series*

The *Teen Health Series* contains a wealth of information about a wide variety of medical topics. As the *Series* continues to grow in size and scope, locating the precise information needed by a specific student may become more challenging. To address this concern, information about books within the *Teen Health Series* is included in *A Contents Guide to the Health Reference Series*. The *Contents Guide* presents an extensive list of more than 16,000 diseases, treatments, and other topics of general interest compiled from the Tables of Contents and major index headings from the books of the *Teen Health Series* and *Health Reference Series*. To access *A Contents Guide to the Health Reference Series*, visit www.healthreferenceseries.com.

Our Advisory Board

We would like to thank the following advisory board members for providing guidance to the development of this *Series*:

Medical Consultant

Medical consultation services are provided to the *Teen Health Series* editors by David A. Cooke, M.D. Dr. Cooke is a graduate of Brandeis University, and he received his M.D. degree from the University of Michigan. He completed residency training at the University of Wisconsin Hospital and Clinics. He is board-certified in internal medicine. Dr. Cooke currently works as part of the University of Michigan Health System and practices in Ann Arbor, MI. In his free time, he enjoys writing, science fiction, and spending time with his family.

Part One
Skin Basics

Chapter 1

Why Skin Is So Important

Your skin is your largest organ. If the skin of a typical 150-pound (68-kilogram) adult male were stretched out flat, it would cover about 2 square yards (1.7 square meters) and weigh about 9 pounds (4 kilograms).

Skin protects the network of muscles, bones, nerves, blood vessels, and everything else inside our bodies. Eyelids have the thinnest skin, the soles of our feet the thickest.

Hair is actually a modified type of skin. Hair grows everywhere on the human body except the palms of the hands, soles of the feet, eyelids, and lips. Hair grows more quickly in summer than winter, and more slowly at night than during the day.

Like hair, nails are a type of modified skin—and they're not just for beauty. Nails protect the sensitive tips of our fingers and toes. Human nails are not necessary for living, but they do provide support for the tips of the fingers and toes, protect them from injury, and aid in picking up small objects. Without them, we'd have a hard time scratching an itch or untying a knot. Nails can be an indicator of a person's general health, and illness often affects their growth.

Skin Basics

Skin is essential to a person's survival. It forms a barrier that prevents harmful substances and microorganisms from entering the body. It protects body tissues against injury. Our skin also controls the loss of life-sustaining fluids like blood and water, helps us regulate body temperature through perspiration, and protects us from the sun's damaging ultraviolet rays.

About This Chapter: From "Skin, Hair, And Nails," May 2012, reprinted with permission from www.kidshealth .org. This information was provided by KidsHealth®, one of the largest resources online for medically reviewed health information written for parents, kids, and teens. For more articles like this, visit www.KidsHealth.org, or www.TeensHealth.org. Copyright © 1995-2012 The Nemours Foundation. All rights reserved.

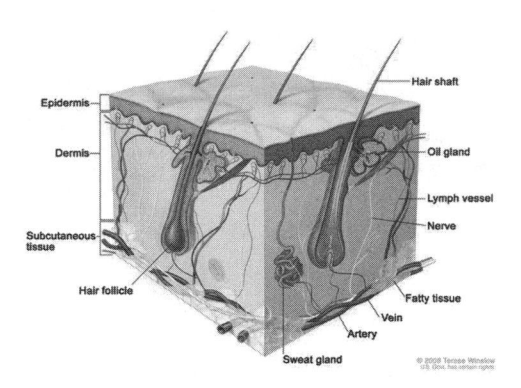

Figure 1.1. Skin anatomy. (Source: © 2008 Terese Winslow, U.S. Govt. has certain rights.)

Without the nerve cells in our skin, we couldn't feel warmth, cold, or other sensations. Our skin can also respond to situations and emotions: Muscles in the skin called **erector pili** contract to make the hairs on our skin stand up straight (goosebumps) when we are cold or frightened—for insulation and protection.

Every square inch of skin contains thousands of cells and hundreds of sweat glands, oil glands, nerve endings, and blood vessels. Skin is made up of three layers: the **epidermis** (pronounced: ep-ih-**dur**-mis), **dermis,** and the **subcutaneous** (pronounced: sub-kyoo-**tay**-nee-us) **tissue.**

Can fingerprints wear off?

No. Even if you injure the skin of your fingers, your fingerprints grow back as they were. Why? Because the dermal papillae—which are responsible for creating your fingerprints—are not in the top layer of your fingertips (epidermis). The dermal papillae are like tiny pegs in the dermis, a deeper skin layer. The papillae poke up from the dermis and are protected by the epidermis, creating the ridges of your fingerprints.

Source: Nemours Foundation, 2012

Skin Cells And Layers

The upper layer of our skin, the epidermis, is the tough, protective outer layer. It is about as thick as a sheet of paper over most parts of the body. The epidermis has four layers of cells that are constantly flaking off and being renewed. In these four layers are three special types of cells:

- **Melanocytes** (pronounced: meh-**lah**-nuh-sites) produce **melanin**, the pigment that give skin its color. All people have roughly the same number of melanocytes; those of dark-skinned people produce more melanin. Exposure to sunlight increases the production of melanin, which is why people get suntanned or freckled.

- **Keratinocyte**s (pronounced: ker-uh-**tih**-no-sites) produce **keratin**, a type of protein basic component of hair and nails. Keratin is also found in skin cells in the skin's outer layer, where it helps create a protective barrier.

- **Langerhans** (pronounced: **lahng**-ur-hanz) **cells** help protect the body against infection.

Because the cells in the epidermis are completely replaced about every 28 days, cuts and scrapes heal quickly.

Below the epidermis is the next layer of our skin, the **dermis,** which is made up of blood vessels, nerve endings, and connective tissue. The dermis nourishes the epidermis.

Without certain molecules in the dermis, our skin wouldn't stretch when we bend or reposition itself when we straighten up. These two types of fibers in the dermis, **collagen** and **elastin**, help the skin stretch and reposition itself when we move. Collagen is strong and hard to stretch and elastin, as its name suggests, is elastic. In older people, some of the elastin-containing fibers degenerate, which is one reason why the skin looks wrinkled (most wrinkles are caused by sun exposure, though!).

The dermis also contains a person's sebaceous glands. These glands, which surround and empty into our hair follicles and pores, produce an oil called **sebum** (pronounced: **see**-bum) that lubricates the skin and hair. Sebaceous glands are found mostly in the skin on the face, upper back, shoulders, and chest.

Most of the time, the sebaceous glands make the right amount of sebum. As a person's body begins to mature and develop during the teenage years, though, hormones stimulate the sebaceous glands to make more sebum. This can lead to acne when pores become clogged by too much sebum and too many dead skin cells. Later in life, these glands produce less sebum, which contributes to dry skin in older people.

The bottom layer of our skin, the **subcutaneous tissue**, is made up of connective tissue, sweat glands, blood vessels, and cells that store fat. This layer helps protect the body from blows and other injuries and helps it hold in body heat.

There are two types of sweat-producing glands. The **eccrine** (pronounced: **eh**-krun) **glands** are found everywhere in our bodies, although they are mostly in the forehead, palms, and soles of the feet. By producing sweat, these glands help regulate body temperature, and waste products are excreted through them.

The other type of sweat-producing gland, **the apocrine glands,** develop at puberty and are concentrated in the armpits and pubic region. The sweat from the apocrine glands is thicker than that produced by the eccrine glands. Although this sweat doesn't smell, when it mixes with bacteria on the skin's surface, it can cause body odor.

A normal, healthy adult secretes about one pint (about half a liter) of sweat daily, but this may be increased by physical activity, fever, or a hot environment.

Hair Basics

The hair on our heads isn't just there for looks. It keeps us warm by preserving heat. The hair in our nose, ears, and around our eyes protects these sensitive areas of the body from dust and other small particles. Eyebrows and eyelashes protect our eyes by decreasing the amount of light and particles that go into them. The fine hair that covers our bodies provides warmth and protects our skin. Hair also cushions the body against injury.

What's It Mean?

Dermis: The middle layer of skin that contains blood vessels, nerve endings, oil glands, and sweat glands. It also contains elastin and collagen, which allow skin to stretch and stay strong.

Epidermis: The top layer of your skin—the part you can see.

Glands: Parts of the skin that release substances including oil (sebum) and sweat.

Keratin: The protein that forms your hair and nails and also helps protect your skin.

Melanin: The pigment that gives your skin its color.

Sebum: Oil produced in the skin to keep skin and hair and hair lubricated, waterproof and protected. Too much sebum can make skin oily (common in teens) and too little can make skin dry (often seen as older people).

Subcutaneous Tissue: The third and bottom layer of skin that mostly contains fat. It helps keeps your body warm and acts as a shock absorber.

—LE

Why do people get goosebumps?

You get goosebumps because your skin is covered with hair. When you get cold, the muscles attached to each hair get tight in an attempt to keep you warm. Those muscles pull your hair and skin up into the air.

Source: Nemours Foundation, 2012

Human hair consists of the **hair shaft,** which projects from the skin's surface, and the **root,** a soft thickened bulb at the base of the hair embedded in the skin. The root ends in the hair bulb. The **hair bulb** sits in a sac-like pit in the skin called the **follicle,** from which the hair grows.

At the bottom of the follicle is the **papilla,** where hair growth actually takes place. The papilla contains an artery that nourishes the root of the hair. As cells multiply and produce keratin to harden the structure, they are pushed up the follicle and through the skin's surface as a shaft of hair. Each hair has three layers: the **medulla** at the center, which is soft; the **cortex,** which surrounds the medulla and is the main part of the hair; and the **cuticle,** the hard outer layer that protects the shaft.

Hair grows by forming new cells at the base of the root. These cells multiply to form a rod of tissue in the skin. The rods of cells move upward through the skin as new cells form beneath them. As they move up, they are cut off from their supply of nourishment and start to form a hard protein called keratin in a process called **keratinization** (pronounced: ker-uh-tuh-nuh-**zay**-shun). As this process occurs, the hair cells die. The dead cells and keratin form the shaft of the hair.

Each hair grows about ¼ inch (about 6 millimeters) every month and keeps on growing for up to six years. The hair then falls out and another grows in its place. The length of a person's hair depends on the length of the growing phase of the follicle. Follicles are active for two to six years; they rest for about three months after that. A person becomes bald if the scalp follicles become inactive and no longer produce new hair. Thick hair grows out of large follicles; narrow follicles produce thin hair.

The color of a person's hair is determined by the amount and distribution of melanin in the cortex of each hair (the same melanin that's found in the epidermis). Hair also contains a yellow-red pigment; people who have blonde or red hair have only a small amount of melanin in their hair. Hair becomes gray when people age because pigment no longer forms.

All About Nails

Nails grow out of deep folds in the skin of the fingers and toes. As epidermal cells below the nail root move up to the surface of the skin, they increase in number, and those closest to the nail root become flattened and pressed tightly together. Each cell is transformed into a thin plate; these plates are piled in layers to form the nail. As with hair, nails are formed by **keratinization.** When the nail cells accumulate, the nail is pushed forward.

The skin below the nail is called the **matrix.** The larger part of the nail, the **nail plate,** looks pink because of the network of tiny blood vessels in the underlying dermis. The whitish crescent-shaped area at the base of the nail is called the **lunula.**

Fingernails grow about three or four times as quickly as toenails. Like hair, nails grow more rapidly in summer than in winter. If a nail is torn off, it will regrow if the matrix is not severely injured. White spots on the nail are sometimes due to temporary changes in growth rate.

What do white spots on your fingernails mean?

The white spots on fingernails are evidence of some trauma that occurred while that part of the nail was growing under the surface of the skin. In other words, if you pinched your finger in a door, that pinch might leave a mark. But you won't see that effect on your fingernail until that part of the nail grows above your cuticle.

Source: Nemours Foundation, 2012

Skin Problems

Some of the things that can affect the skin, nails, and hair are described below.

Dermatitis

Medical experts use the term **dermatitis** (pronounced: dur-mah-**ty**-tus) to refer to any inflammation that might be associated with swelling, itching, and redness of the skin. There are many types of dermatitis, including:

- **Atopic dermatitis** is also called eczema. It's a common, hereditary dermatitis that causes an itchy rash primarily on the face, trunk, arms, and legs. It commonly develops in infancy, but can also appear in early childhood. It may be associated with allergic diseases such as asthma or food, seasonal, or environmental allergies.

- **Contact dermatitis** occurs when the skin comes into contact with an irritating substance or a substance that a person is allergic to. The best-known cause of contact dermatitis is poison ivy. But lots of other things cause contact dermatitis, including chemicals found in laundry detergent, cosmetics, and perfumes, and metals like jewelry, nickel plating on a belt buckle, or the back of the buttons on your jeans.

- **Seborrheic dermatitis**, an oily rash on the scalp, face, chest, and back, is related to an overproduction of sebum from the sebaceous glands. This condition is common in teens.

Bacterial Skin Infections

- **Impetigo:** Impetigo (pronounced: im-puh-**ty**-go) is a bacterial infection that results in a honey-colored, crusty rash, often on the face near the mouth and nose.

- **Cellulitis:** Cellulitis (pronounced: sell-yuh-ly-tus) is an infection of the skin and subcutaneous tissue that typically occurs when bacteria are introduced through a puncture, bite, or other break in the skin. The cellulitic area is usually warm and tender and has some redness.

- **Streptococcal And Staphylococcal Infections:** These two kinds of bacteria are the main causes of cellulitis and impetigo. Certain types of these bacteria are also responsible for distinctive rashes on the skin, including the rashes associated with scarlet fever and toxic shock syndrome.

Fungal Infections Of The Skin And Nails

- **Candidal Dermatitis:** A warm, moist environment, such as that found in the folds of the skin in the diaper area of infants, is perfect for growth of the yeast *Candida*. Yeast infections of the skin in older children, teens, and adults are less common

- **Tinea Infection (Ringworm):** Ringworm, which isn't a worm at all, is a fungus infection that can affect the skin, nails, or scalp. Tinea (pronounced: **tih**-nee-uh) fungi can infect the skin and related tissues of the body. The medical name for ringworm of the scalp is tinea capitis; ringworm of the body is called tinea corporis; and ringworm of the nails is called tinea unguium. With tinea corporis, the fungi can cause scaly, ring-like lesions anywhere on the body.

- **Tinea Pedis (Athlete's Foot):** This infection of the feet is caused by the same types of fungi (called dermatophytes) that cause ringworm. Athlete's foot is commonly found in adolescents and is more likely to occur during warm weather.

Other Skin Problems

- **Parasitic Infestations:** Parasites (usually tiny insects or worms) can feed on or burrow into the skin, often resulting in an itchy rash. Scabies and lice are examples of parasitic infestations. Both are contagious—meaning they can be easily caught from other people.

- **Viral Infections:** Many viruses cause characteristic rashes on the skin, including **varicella** (pronounced: var-ih-**seh**-luh), the virus that causes chicken pox and shingles; herpes simplex, which causes cold sores; human papillomavirus (HPV), the virus that causes warts; and a host of others.

- **Acne (Acne Vulgaris):** Acne is the single most common skin condition in teens. Some degree of acne is seen in 85 percent of adolescents, and nearly all teens have the occasional pimple, blackhead, or whitehead.

- **Skin Cancer:** Skin cancer is rare in children and teens, but good sun protection habits established during these years can help prevent skin cancers like **melanoma** (pronounced: meh-luh-**no**-ma, a serious form of skin cancer that can spread to other parts of the body) later in life, especially among fair-skinned people who sunburn easily.

In addition to these diseases and conditions, the skin can be injured in a number of ways. Minor scrapes, cuts, and bruises heal quickly on their own, but other injuries—severe cuts and burns, for example—require medical treatment.

Disorders Of The Scalp And Hair

- **Tinea capitis,** a type of ringworm, is a fungal infection that forms a scaly, ring-like lesion in the scalp. It's contagious and common among school-age children.

- **Alopecia** (pronounced: ah-luh-**pee**-sha) is an area of hair loss. Ringworm is a common cause of temporary alopecia in children. Alopecia can also be caused by tight braiding that pulls on the hair roots (this condition is called **traction alopecia**). Alopecia areata (where a person's hair falls out in round or oval patches on the scalp) is a less common condition that can sometimes affect teens.

Chapter 2

Freckles And Brown Spots

Freckles

Freckles are small flat brown marks arising on the face and other sun exposed areas. They are most often seen in fair-skinned people, especially those with red hair, but they are an inherited characteristic that sometimes affects darker skin types as well.

The medical term for this type of freckle is "ephelis" (plural "ephelides"). The color is due to pigment accumulating in the skin cells (keratinocytes).

Skin pigment (melanin) is made by cells called melanocytes. They don't produce much melanin during the winter months, but produce more when exposed to the sun. The melanin is diffused into the surrounding skin cells, called keratinocytes. The color of ephelides is due to localized accumulation of melanin in keratinocytes.

Ephelides are more prominent in summer but fade considerably or disappear in winter as the keratinocytes are replaced by new cells.

As the person ages this type of freckle generally become less noticeable. Apart from sun protection, no particular treatment is necessary.

Lentigines

Larger flat brown spots on the face and hands arising in middle age also result from sun damage exposure. Unlike freckles they tend to persist for long periods and don't disappear in

About This Chapter: "Brown Spots and Freckles," reprinted with permission from DermNet NZ, the web site of the New Zealand Dermatological Society. Visit www.dermnetnz.org for patient information about skin diseases, conditions, and treatment. © 2013 New Zealand Dermatological Society. All rights reserved.

the winter (though they may fade). Commonly known as age spots or liver spots, the correct term for a single lesion is "solar lentigo" (plural "lentigines").

Lentigines are common in those with fair skin but are also frequently seen in those who tan easily or have naturally dark skin. Lentigines are due to localized proliferation of melanocytes.

It is important to distinguish the harmless solar lentigo from an early malignant melanoma, the "lentigo maligna." If the freckle has arisen recently, is made up of more than one color or has irregular borders, or if you have any doubts, see your dermatologist for advice.

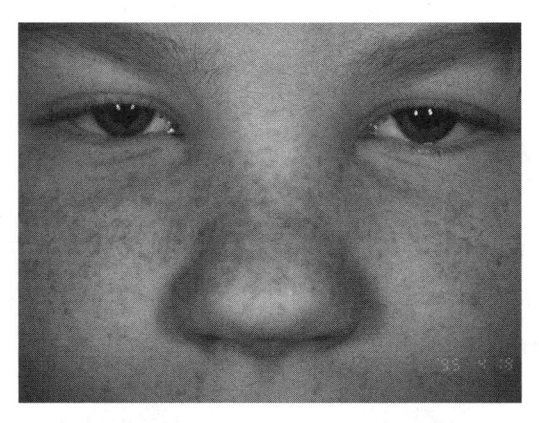

Figure 2.1. Freckles (Source © 2013 New Zealand Dermatological Society).

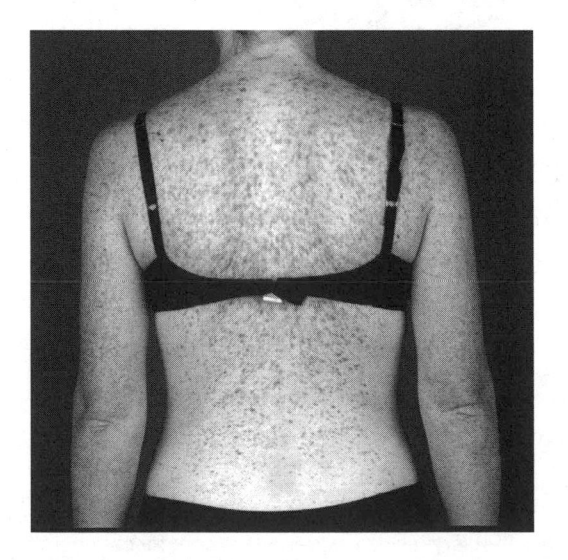

Figure 2.2. Lentigines (Source © 2013 New Zealand Dermatological Society).

Other Brown Marks

If the brown marks are scaly, they may be solar keratoses (sun damage) or seborrheic keratoses (senile warts). In this case there is a proliferation of keratinocytes.

Treatment Of Brown Marks

Brown marks may fade with careful sun protection, broad-spectrum sunscreen applied daily for nine months of the year. Regular applications of anti-aging or "fading" creams may also help. These may contain hydroquinone, or antioxidants such as:

- alpha hydroxy acids;
- vitamin C;
- retinoids;
- azelaic acid.

However, brown marks may be removed more rapidly and effectively by chemical peels, cryotherapy, or certain pigment lasers that target melanin in the skin. Multiple treatments may be necessary.

Suitable green-light devices include:

- flashlamp-pulsed tunable dye laser;
- frequency doubled Q-switched Nd:YAG laser (neodynium:yttrium-aluminium-garnet);
- KTP laser;
- Krypton laser;
- copper bromide laser.

Suitable red light devices include:

- Q-switched alexandrite;
- Q-switched ruby.

Intense pulsed light has a similar effect. Carbon dioxide and erbium:YAG lasers vaporize the surface skin thus removing the pigmented lesions. A fractional laser may also be effective.

Results are variable but sometimes very impressive with minimal risk of scarring.

With superficial resurfacing techniques, there is minimal discomfort and no down-time but several treatments are often necessary. Unfortunately the treatment occasionally makes the pigmentation worse. Continued careful sun protection is essential, because the pigmentation is likely to recur next summer.

Follow-Up

If there is any doubt whether a brown mark may be a cancer, your doctor may choose to observe the lesion (e.g., with mole mapping or photography) or excise it for pathological examination.

Chapter 3

Blushing

When people are afraid, angry, anxious, or scared, their body makes extra adrenalin so that they can fight or run away (depending on what is needed). Our bodies still work in the same way now as they did thousands of years ago, but our societies have changed a lot. Nowadays fighting or running may not be possible or useful, but the extra adrenalin is still made.

Some of the effects of the extra adrenalin are:

- The heart beats faster and more strongly.

- Blood pressure rises and blood vessels dilate (get larger) so that extra blood, carrying oxygen and glucose for energy, can go to muscles.

- Breathing becomes deeper and faster.

As a result, blood vessels in the face and neck also dilate, causing flushing (blushing) and often increased sweating.

When does blushing happen?

Almost everyone blushes when they are angry, anxious, scared, or embarrassed.

- Situations where people most commonly blush are those where the person has to do something when a lot of people will be watching them. Their body prepares them to fight or run away, but they have to stand still and "perform." Many people are very anxious when they have to speak in front of a class or a larger audience.

About This Chapter: Reprinted with permission from Women's and Children's Health Network (www.cyh.com). © 2012 Government of South Australia.

- Other people blush when something that embarrasses them happens, such as when their friends ask about their boyfriend or girlfriend.

- Walking into a new class, meeting friends when you have to walk in alone, being asked a question and everyone looking at you are all situations when everyone can feel nervous or clumsy.

If the person has pale skin, the blushing can be easy to see, although people with darker skin also blush.

What do people think?

If people notice that another person is blushing they might think:

- That person is being very brave doing something that is hard.

- That person is angry, and maybe there is something that can be done to help the person.

- That person is embarrassed by what is happening—how can we help?

- That I blush in the same situation.

There may be some unkind people who think it is funny, but most people do not think this way. Actually most people do not notice if someone is blushing. They are thinking about what they themselves are doing and perhaps about how hard it is going to be to also have to talk in front of the class when it is their turn. They often do not notice how hard it is for someone else.

What can be done about blushing?

Blushing is a natural response which involves the whole body, not just your face and neck, and trying to stop it by using any medicines is not a good idea.

- You could try some self-talk, such as:

  - People will think that I am brave when they can see that I am anxious.

  - Most people won't notice that I am blushing.

  - So, I'm blushing again—well, I can't do anything about, it so I just have to carry on.

- You could practice talking in front of other people so that you do not feel so anxious.

- You could practice what it is that you will have to do in front of a special friend or in front of the mirror, so that you can be confident that what you are saying makes sense and is well organized.

- You could politely ask other people not to talk about things that embarrass you.

- You could laugh it off and say, "Oh you're making me blush!"

- You could make sure that you are wearing a good deodorant so that you don't feel too embarrassed if you also start to sweat a lot!

If you are going to have to do something that you feel extremely anxious about, have a talk with your doctor, as there may be something that could help you get through that one event.

If you are not so anxious, you might not blush as much—but really, the medicine is for the anxiety, not for the blushing.

Chapter 4

Ethnicity And Skin

Frequently Asked Questions

What does the term, "ethnic skin" mean?

Ethnic skin encompasses a wide variety of skin types, including, but not limited to: African Americans, Asians, Latinos, Native Americans, Mediterranean, and people of mixed ethnicities.

How is ethnic skin different from Caucasian skin?

Ethnic skin, or skin of color, has more melanin than Caucasian skin, in varying degrees, depending upon the skin type and the individual. There are both benefits and risks associated with darker pigmented skin. Due to the higher amount of melanin, the skin may appear up to 10 years younger than that of a Caucasian the same age. The extra melanin also provides some added, although not fully adequate, protection for ultraviolet (UV) damage to the skin.

There are special risk factors unique to ethnic skin, which have to do with the extra melanin, which can create various pigmentation disorders, such as hyperpigmentation, post-inflammatory hyperpigmentation (PIH), acne scarring, keloids, melasma, and vitiligo.

About This Chapter: The information in this chapter is reprinted with permission from: "America's Ethnic Skin: Frequently Asked Questions," "Acne/Post-Inflammatory Hyperpigmentation," by Mary Lupo, MD, FAAD, "Rosacea in Skin of Color," by Valerie D. Callender, MD, FAAD, and "Sun Protection for Ethnic Skin Types," by Henry W. Lim, MD, FAAD, Suzanne Connolly, MD, FAAD, and Sandra Read, MD, FAAD. All documents © 2009 Women's Dermatologic Society. All rights reserved. For additional information, visit http://www.womensderm.org.

Is it true that darker skin types need sun protection if they have the extra melanin as a built-in SPF?

Yes, it is essential for all skin types, including people with skin of color, to protect their skin from harmful ultraviolet radiation. Even though darker skin types may have a "built-in" SPF of between 8–13, depending upon the amount of pigment in the skin, that is still not enough to properly guard against the sun's harmful rays.

What is the proper way to for people with ethnic skin to use sunscreen?

It is recommended to use a broad-spectrum (UVA/UVB) sunscreen with a sun protection factor (SPF) of 15 or higher. Broad-spectrum means protection from the UVA rays (which are associated with aging) and UVB rays (which are associated with burns). Sunscreen needs to be applied properly and regularly. In addition, people should wear a wide-brimmed hat, sunglasses, and avoid the sun during peak hours (10 a.m. – 4 p.m.)

How can I find a dermatologist experienced in treating ethnic skin?

To find a dermatologist, you may visit:

http://www.aad.org/findaderm/ (and type in your zip code)

http://www.womensderm.org/find/ (and type in your zip code)

To find out if a doctor is board-certified, you may visit:

http://www.abderm.org/

It is advisable to get personal referrals and check to be sure that the dermatologist is well-experienced in treating darker skin types.

Acne/Post-Inflammatory Hyperpigmentation

Acne can have various causes. Heredity, hormonal irregularities, stress, and pore-clogging cosmetics and hair products are the most common. If there is an underlying condition, such as polycystic ovary syndrome, it is important to get medical treatment to correct it.

There are many presentations of acne. Papules, pustules, blackheads, whiteheads, nodules, and cysts can be seen. Lesions are caused by blockage of the pores resulting in a build-up of oil and bacteria. The digestion of the oil by the bacteria results in inflammation. Picking and squeezing can further increase the inflammation.

Dermatologists adjust their treatment of acne in darker skin individuals. Care must be taken to avoid unnecessary irritation that can increase post-inflammatory hyperpigmentation. Topical creams are used to improve the turnover of skin cells (exfoliate), and to decrease bacteria. Oral antibiotics are often beneficial. In severe or stubborn cases, oral retinoids can be used. Oral contraceptives and other male hormone blocking agents are sometimes useful. As with all medications, side effects are possible and your prescribing dermatologist will discuss the relative risks and benefits.

Post-inflammatory hyperpigmentation is very common among darker-skin ethnic groups. Burns, bites, and acne are typical causes. The inflammation causes a stimulation of pigment production. If the skin is injured into the deeper level, the pigment will appear darker and be even more resistant to treatment.

Post-inflammatory hyperpigmentation is a common, yet difficult problem to treat. Topical bleaching agents, retinoids, and some topical anti-inflammatory agents are helpful. Light chemical peels and microdermabrasion have been found to be safe and effective. Risks and benefits of all procedures should be discussed with your dermatologist.

Always seek the advice of a board certified dermatologist for the best information on the care and treatment of your skin.

Rosacea In Skin Of Color

Rosacea, or commonly referred to as "adult acne," is a common skin disorder that affects approximately 14 million Americans. The exact cause of rosacea is unknown; however there are several trigger factors that are associated with rosacea flares. These include hot drinks, spicy foods, caffeine, and alcoholic drinks. Heat and exercise can also worsen rosacea.

Rosacea occurs mainly on the central areas of the face which includes the cheeks, forehead, chin, and nose. Initially the skin may show a tendency to flush easily and it gradually progresses to persistent redness.

As the condition worsens, tiny blood vessels appear on the skin surface along with red pimples (some with pus inside) that can be confused with acne; but unlike acne, rosacea does not cause blackheads and whiteheads. If left untreated, rosacea can worsen and develop into rhinophyma, a condition where the oil glands of the nose and cheeks enlarge and the skin becomes red, thickened, and lumpy. This more advanced form of rosacea occurs mainly in men. In fact, W.C. Fields was probably the most famous sufferer of rhinophyma.

Rosacea occurs in all races and ethnicities, including people of color. An important difference between light and dark skin is that people of color are more likely to develop hypopigmentation (light spots) or hyperpigmentation (dark spots), from inflammation or any kind of skin trauma. Therefore, inflamed red pimples, which are often seen in rosacea sufferers, can lead to changes in the skin pigmentation in the affected areas.

Rosacea may also affect the eyes. In fact, about 50 percent of people have eye involvement and may experience redness, burning, and irritation of the eyes, a condition called conjunctivitis. If left untreated, the eye problems can lead to more serious complications. Therefore, ophthalmologists or eye doctors must also be aware of the occurrence of rosacea.

The best treatment for rosacea starts with going to a dermatologist to identify the condition early on. Current treatments your dermatologist might recommend include topical and oral antibiotics and products containing sodium sulfacetamide or azelaic acid.

Other recommendations include strict avoidance of rosacea's triggering factors and sun protection with sunscreens/sunblocks that are broad-spectrum with a SPF 15 and higher.

The key to successful rosacea management is early diagnosis and combination therapy.

Sun Protection For Ethnic Skin Types

- Ultraviolet (UV) radiation from the sun, or from artificial light sources, can be divided into longer wavelength UVA, which causes tanning and wrinkling of the skin, and shorter wavelength UVB, which causes sunburn.

- Remember: "A" in UVA stands for skin aging, "B" in UVB for sunburn.

- SPF (sun protection factor) is a reflection on how well the sunscreen product protects the skin from redness caused by sun exposure. It is therefore an assessment of protection against the effect of UVB.

- Because of the propensity for tanning, minor blemishes in ethnic skin types can become quite dark and noticeable, primarily because of the tanning response upon exposure to sunlight.

- Therefore, it is important for ethnic skin types to select good broad-spectrum sunscreens that protect against the effect of UVB and UVA. Look for products SPF of 15 or above that contain avobenzone (Parsol 1789), ecamsule (Mexoryl SX), titanium dioxide, and/or zinc oxide.

- The use of sunscreens is only one component of photoprotection. Proper photoprotection should include seeking shade during the peak UV hours (10 a.m. to 4 p.m.), the use of protective clothing, wide-brimmed hat, sunscreens, and sunglasses.

- For those concerned about vitamin D insufficiency, balanced diet, vitamin D fortified food and drink, and vitamin D3 supplement can be considered.

Chapter 5

Healthy Body Image And Self-Esteem For Teens With Facial Differences

If you have a scar, birthmark, or uniquely shaped face, you probably know how hard it can be to look different from everyone else. You might be reminded of that difference every time you look in the mirror or see someone staring in your direction. Major differences in appearance due to burns, birth defects, or other diseases and disorders can contribute to negative body image and low self-esteem. The effects of body image on self-esteem can be especially powerful during the teenage years. Although it's perfectly normal to have negative thoughts and feelings towards your facial difference, finding ways to be positive is the key to building a healthy body image and good self-esteem.

What is body image?

Body image is based on your thoughts and feelings about the way your body looks. Sometimes, the way you think other people are judging your appearance can influence your body image. Poor body image comes from negative thoughts and feelings about your appearance. Healthy body image is made up of thoughts and feelings that are positive. Body image is a major factor in self-esteem.

What is self-esteem?

Self-esteem relates to the way you think and feel about yourself as a person. This includes how you recognize or appreciate your individual character, qualities, skills, and accomplishments. As with body image, self-esteem can also be based on how you *think* other people look at you as a person. People who have low self-esteem may not feel confident about themselves or how they look. It's often hard for them to see that they are an important and capable person. People with good self-esteem have a positive and confident attitude about their body and mind, and can recognize their strengths as well as personal value and worth.

Remember

- It can be hard to look different than everyone else.
- Finding ways to have a healthy body image is important.
- Be confident in yourself.

Why is good self-esteem important?

Good self-esteem is important for everyone because it helps you keep a positive outlook on life, and makes you feel proud of the person you are—on the inside and outside. Most teens with good self-esteem find life much more enjoyable. They tend to have better relationships with their peers and with adults, find it easier to deal with mistakes or disappointments, and are more likely to stick with a task until they succeed.

Good self-esteem gives you:

- The courage to try new things
- The power to believe in yourself
- The confidence to make healthy choices for your mind and body

How is my self-esteem affected by my facial difference?

It's common to look at other people and compare your own appearance. For example, you might compare facial features such as your nose, lips, eyes, or hair. A normal part of having a facial difference is feeling like you are not as attractive as other people. Feeling unattractive or different can keep you from meeting new people and trying new things. If you start to feel bad about your facial difference, you may begin to feel bad about other parts of yourself as well.

Treating yourself with respect and realizing that every part of you is worth caring for and protecting will help you keep a positive attitude towards yourself. Building good self-esteem can take a long time and is not always easy, but knowing that you can improve your self-esteem is the first step.

How do other people's reactions to my facial difference affect my self-esteem?

Just like many other teens with facial differences, you may also have trouble dealing with people who stare, question, or make comments about your appearance. Anyone (with or without a facial difference) often feels uncomfortable if they are being stared at. These situations can make it difficult to meet new people, make friends, try out for sports teams, join clubs, and even apply for a job. It's hard to have pride and confidence if you feel like most social interactions leave you feeling bad about yourself. It's important to understand that you have the power to answer questions or respond to comments with confidence, and not let another person's words or stares lower your self-esteem.

Should I take it personally when other people stare or ask questions about my facial difference?

It's easy to think that when other people are staring at you they are negatively judging your appearance, but most of the time people are not judging you as a person—they are simply being curious. Others may ask questions out of care and concern, and are not trying to be rude. Someone who sees you for the first time knows only one thing about you: what you look like. Your personality is not based on looks, so you shouldn't take a stranger's questions or stares personally, because they don't know anything else about you. When someone stares or asks questions, see it as a chance to increase their awareness about your facial difference. Most people have little knowledge about facial differences and haven't met anyone who has them. You can clear up any misunderstandings they may have about you so that they don't assume anything that isn't true.

What are some positive or helpful ways to respond when people stare, comment, or ask questions?

It can be very frustrating when other people comment or stare, but if you know what to say and feel confident about yourself, the curiosity of others won't feel so uncomfortable. You can try something called **P.Y.A**, which stands for "**P**repare **Y**our **A**nswer." First, think about some of the possible questions you might be asked. Next, write a few short answers about what your facial difference is and maybe why you have it. You might realize that you don't know a lot about your condition, so look through some books, check out reliable websites, and talk with your healthcare provider to learn as much as you can.

Here are some tips to remember when thinking about what to say:

- **Speak confidently.** Show others that you have no reason to be ashamed or embarrassed.

- **Consider the age of the person you are talking to.** For example: If you have a cleft lip, a young child probably won't understand what that means. You will need to explain it with words they will understand, such as: "My mouth wasn't finished growing when I was born."

- **Don't describe your condition with negative words.** If you use words like "ugly" or "stupid" and say "I have an ugly/stupid scar," this will only confirm any negative thoughts others may have, and it can become harder for you to build good self-esteem.

- **Share only what you are comfortable sharing.** If there are details that you would rather not share with strangers it's OK to politely end the conversation by saying something such as, "I'm not comfortable answering your question."

Here are some sample situations and possible ways to respond:

- **Situation #1:** You've been in a burn accident that left scars covering most of your face. When you try out for a sports team at school, the coach wonders if you will be able to participate without limitations.

  Your Response: "The scars on my face don't affect my ability to play sports. I'm still a strong and competitive athlete."

- **Situation #2:** You're at a friend's house, and her younger sister who is about four or five years old notices that you have a red patch of skin on your face (your strawberry birthmark) and asks: "What's wrong with your face?"

  Your Response: Smile and gently explain, "My face looks different because I was born with something that makes my skin this color. Sometimes things can change how your skin looks."

- **Situation #3:** You have a syndrome that caused the shape of your face to develop differently. While you are on the bus, a teen sitting across from you begins to stare.

  Your Response: Make eye contact, smile, and simply say "Hi!" You could also say something friendly, such as complimenting their outfit.

Remember that there is so much more to you than just physical appearance. Respond and interact with people in a way that lets them see your inner qualities too. Find ways to let your skills or talents shine. Show that you have hobbies, interests, likes, and dislikes just like everyone else.

What if someone asks about my facial difference but I just don't feel like talking about it?

That's OK! *You* are in control of the conversation and have the right to say that you would rather not answer their question. It can be especially uncomfortable when someone questions you in a public place or in the presence of other curious people where it suddenly feels like you have an audience. Changing the subject of the conversation might help the other person know that you don't feel like talking. If people are staring, it's OK to look in another direction or walk away.

Is there anything I can do if I feel frustrated?

If you feel frustrated, or too annoyed or upset to talk, try going for a walk or a run, listen to music, or participate in a fun activity with someone you enjoy being with. Sometimes expressing how you feel can actually be more helpful than keeping feelings to yourself. Talk with a close friend or relative who you trust, and who can offer encouragement and support. It can also be comforting to talk with other teens that may be going through similar experiences.

> If you are feeling very sad and discouraged most of the time, and can't seem to find ways to feel better about yourself, it is important to contact your healthcare provider or counselor. They can help you to find ways to cope.

What can I do to build self-confidence in the way I look?

Since your facial difference is only one aspect of your appearance, try and concentrate on feeling good about your whole body. There are many ways to help boost self-confidence, such as finding a flattering outfit to wear, getting a new hairstyle, or simply eating nutritious foods and exercising. One of the best ways to feel good about your body is to know that you have a healthy one! You may not have control over your facial difference, but you do have the power to keep a positive attitude about yourself.

What are some ways to keep a positive attitude?

You can keep a positive attitude by defining an identity for yourself that is not based on looks or negative things other people may say.

Some ways you can develop good self-esteem and keep a positive attitude are:

- **Focusing on the good things you do** and spending time concentrating on your unique qualities.

- **Focusing on your education.** Learning gives you the power to make a difference in your life and in the lives of others.

- **Participating in a variety of sports or activities.** This can be a great way to stay healthy and fit, which adds to a positive body image.

- **Taking up a new hobby, or learning to play an instrument.** Have you ever wanted to play the guitar? Maybe you want to learn how to play chess. Take time to find your hidden talents!

- **Setting and reaching new goals.** Having something to look forward to can give you a sense of pride and help you work through different challenges throughout your life.

- **Being an inspiration to others.** If you've thought of your own ways to cope with social situations and find confidence, you may find it rewarding to share advice and offer encouragement to others.

Building a healthy body image and good self-esteem can be hard work because it takes time to become confident with your appearance. As you work to improve your body image, you will experience self-acceptance and learn to recognize the qualities, skills, and talents that make you special.

Chapter 6

How Smoking Affects The Way You Look

Introduction

Tobacco smoking seriously affects internal organs, particularly the heart and lungs, but it also affects a person's appearance.

While these changes are generally not as life threatening as heart and lung disease, they can, nevertheless, increase the risk of more serious disorders and have a noticeable ageing effect on the body.

Smoking And Skin

The skin is affected by tobacco smoke in at least two ways. Firstly, tobacco smoke released into the environment has a drying effect on the skin's surface. Secondly, because smoking restricts blood vessels, it reduces the amount of blood flowing to the skin, thus depleting the skin of oxygen and essential nutrients.

Some research suggests that smoking may reduce the body's store of vitamin A, which provides protection against some skin-damaging agents produced by smoking. Another likely explanation is that squinting in response to the irritating nature of the smoke, and the puckering of the mouth when drawing on a cigarette causes wrinkling around the eyes and mouth.

Skin damaged by smoke has a greyish, wasted appearance. Research has shown that the skin-ageing effects of smoking may be due to increased production of an enzyme that breaks down collagen in the skin. Collagen is the main structural protein of the skin which maintains

---

About This Chapter: From "How Smoking Affects The Way You Look," © 2009 Action on Smoking and Health (www.ash.urg.uk). All rights reserved. Reprinted with permission.

elasticity. The more a person smokes, the greater the risk of premature wrinkling. Darkening of the skin around the eyes is also a possible effect of smoking.

Smokers in their 40s often have as many facial wrinkles as nonsmokers in their 60s. In addition to facial wrinkling, smokers may develop hollow cheeks through repeated sucking on cigarettes: This is particularly noticeable in underweight smokers and can cause smokers to look gaunt. A South Korean study of smokers, nonsmokers, and ex-smokers aged 20 to 69 found that the current smokers had a higher degree of facial wrinkling than nonsmokers and ex-smokers. Past smokers who smoked heavily at a younger age revealed less facial wrinkling than current smokers.

The Chief Medical Officer highlighted the link between smoking and wrinkled, damaged skin in his 2003 annual report. The report noted that a smoker's skin can be prematurely aged by between 10 and 20 years and, although the damaging effects of cigarette smoke on the skin are irreversible, further deterioration can be avoided by stopping smoking.

Prolonged smoking causes discoloration of the fingers and fingernails on the hand used to hold cigarettes.

Smoking And Psoriasis

Compared with nonsmokers, smokers have a two to threefold higher risk of developing psoriasis, a chronic skin condition, which, while not life threatening, can be extremely uncomfortable and disfiguring. Some studies have found a dose-response association of smoking and psoriasis, that is, the risk of the disease increases the longer a person continues to smoke. Smoking also appears to be more strongly associated with psoriasis among women than among men. Smoking may cause as many as one-quarter of all psoriasis cases and may also contribute to as many as half of the cases of palmoplantar pustulosis, a skin disease involving the hands and feet, that some experts view as a form of psoriasis.

Smoking And Weight

When people stop smoking, they usually put on weight. Although this is often a cause for concern, the average weight gain is around 2 to 3 kilograms (kg) (about 4.4 to 6.6 pounds) and may be temporary. Although the reasons for weight gain are not fully understood, it has been partly explained by the fact that smoking increases the body's metabolic rate—that is, the rate at which calories are burned up. In addition, nicotine may act as an appetite suppressant so that when smokers quit an increase in appetite leads to an increase in calorie intake. The effect of nicotine on metabolic rate may also explain why smokers tend to weigh less than nonsmokers.

Experts believe that one way smoking raises metabolic rate is by stimulating the nervous system to produce catecholamines (hormones which cause the heart to beat faster), thus making the body burn more calories. Nicotine also produces more thermogenesis, the process by which the body produces heat. This too, causes the body to use up more calories.

However, a smoking-induced increase in metabolic rate only accounts for about half the difference in weight between the average smoker and average nonsmoker. Another likely mechanism is that smoking alters the body-weight set point, that is, the weight towards which a person tends to return despite attempts to gain or lose weight. Smoking appears to lower a person's normal weight and the weight gained on stopping reflects a return to the body's natural weight set point.

Women and girls tend to be more concerned about their weight and body shape than men, and weight control may be influential in causing the higher incidence of smoking among teenage girls. However, post-cessation weight gain can be modified by eating a low-fat, calorie-reduced diet and by moderately increased exercise. One study found that stopping smoking resulted in a net excess weight gain of about 2.4 kg (5.3 pounds) in middle-aged women but that among those women who increased physical activity after stopping smoking, weight gain was between 1.3 kg and 1.8 kg (2.9 and 4 pounds).

While weight gain is common immediately after stopping smoking, in the longer term, ex-smokers weight may return to the comparative weight of someone who has never smoked. A Japanese study examined the relationship between weight gain and the length of time after stopping smoking. Researchers found that although heavy smokers experienced large weight gain and weighed more than never smokers in the few years after smoking cessation, thereafter they lost weight to the never-smoker level. Among former light and moderate smokers, weight was gained up to the never-smoker level but without any further excess gain.

The combination of excess weight and smoking has also been shown to accelerate the ageing process of the body. A study showed that being both overweight and a smoker can age a person by 10 years or more.

Other Effects

Halitosis (bad breath) and stained teeth and gums are perhaps the best-known and most obvious effects of smoking. Tobacco use increases the risk of periodontitis, which results in swollen gums, bad breath and may cause teeth to fall out. Smoking may indeed be responsible for more than half of periodontitis cases among adults.

Smoke can also damage eye blood vessels creating a bloodshot appearance and causing irritation.

Part Two
Acne

Chapter 7

Acne Basics

Why Do I Get Acne?

If you're a teen, chances are pretty good that you have some acne. Almost 8 in 10 teens have acne, along with many adults.

Acne is so common that it's considered a normal part of puberty. But knowing that doesn't always make it easier when you're looking at a big pimple on your face in the mirror. So what is acne, and what can you do about it?

What Is Acne And What Causes It?

Acne is a condition of the skin that shows up as different types of bumps. These bumps can be blackheads, whiteheads, pimples, or cysts. Teens get acne because of the hormonal changes that come with puberty. If your parents had acne as teens, it's more likely that you will, too. The good news is that, for most people, acne goes away almost completely by the time they are out of their teens.

The type of acne that a lot of teens get is called *acne vulgaris* (the meaning of "vulgaris" isn't as bad as it sounds—it means "of the common type"). It usually shows up on the face, neck, shoulders, upper back, and chest.

The hair follicles, or pores, in your skin contain **sebaceous glands** (also called oil glands). These glands make **sebum**, which is an oil that lubricates your hair and skin. Most of the time,

About This Chapter: "Why Do I Get Acne?" January, 2011, reprinted with permission from www.kidshealth .org. This information was provided by KidsHealth®, one of the largest resources online for medically reviewed health information written for parents, kids, and teens. For more articles like this, visit www.KidsHealth.org, or www.TeensHealth.org. Copyright © 1995-2012 The Nemours Foundation. All rights reserved.

the sebaceous glands make the right amount of sebum. As a teen's body begins to mature and develop, though, hormones stimulate the sebaceous glands to make more sebum, and the glands may become overactive. Pores become clogged if there is too much sebum and too many dead skin cells. Bacteria (especially one called *Propionibacterium acnes*) can then get trapped inside the pores and multiply, causing swelling and redness—the start of acne.

If a pore gets clogged up and closes but bulges out from the skin, you're left with a **whitehead**. If a pore gets clogged up but stays open, the top surface can darken and you're left with a **blackhead**. Sometimes the wall of the pore opens, allowing sebum, bacteria, and dead skin cells to make their way under the skin—and you're left with a small, red bump called a **pimple** (sometimes pimples have a pus-filled top from the body's reaction to the bacterial infection).

Clogged pores that open up very deep in the skin can cause **nodules**, which are infected lumps or cysts that are bigger than pimples and can be painful. Occasionally, large cysts that seem like acne may be boils caused by a staph infection.

Acne Myths

There are a few myths out there about things that cause acne—like the one about eating chocolate causing acne. Some people do find that they notice their breakouts get more severe when they eat too much of a certain food, though. If you're one of them, it's worth trying to cut back on that food to see what happens.

Stress doesn't usually cause acne either (although it can make existing acne worse because stress increases sebum production).

Other myths talk about what helps make acne better. Acne isn't really helped by the sun. Although a tan can temporarily make acne look less severe, it won't help it go away permanently—and some people find that the oils their skin produces after being in the sun make their pimples worse.

What Can I Do About Acne?

To help prevent the oil buildup that can contribute to acne, wash your face once or twice a day with a mild soap and warm water. **Don't** scrub your face hard with a washcloth—acne can't be scrubbed away, and scrubbing may actually make it worse by irritating the skin and pores. Try cleansing your face as gently as you can.

If you wear makeup or sunscreen, make sure it's labeled "oil free," "noncomedogenic," or "non-acnegenic." This means it won't clog your pores and contribute to acne. And when you are washing your face, be sure you take the time to remove all of your makeup so it doesn't clog your pores.

If you use hair sprays or gels, try to keep them away from your face, as they can also clog pores. If you have long hair that touches your face, be sure to wash it frequently enough to keep oil away. And if you have an after-school job that puts you in contact with oil—like in a fast-food restaurant or gas station, for example—be sure to wash your face well when you get home. It can also help to wash your face after you've been exercising.

Many over-the-counter lotions and creams containing salicylic acid or benzoyl peroxide are available to help prevent acne and clear it up at the same time. You can experiment with these to see which helps. Be sure to follow the instructions exactly—don't use more than you're supposed to at one time (your skin may get **too** dried out and feel and look worse) and follow any directions to see if you're allergic to it first.

What If I Get Acne Anyway?

Sometimes even though they wash properly and try lotions and oil-free makeup, people get acne anyway—and this is totally normal. In fact, some girls who normally have a handle on their acne may find that it comes out a few days before they get their period. This is called premenstrual acne, and about 7 out of 10 women get it from changes in hormones in the body.

Some teens who have acne can get help from a doctor or dermatologist (a doctor who specializes in skin problems). A doctor may treat the acne with prescription medicines. Depending on the person's acne, this might mean using prescription creams that prevent pimples from forming, taking antibiotics to kill the bacteria that help create pimples, or if the acne is severe, taking stronger medicines such as isotretinoin, or even having minor surgery. Some girls find that birth control pills help to clear up their acne.

If you look in the mirror and see a pimple, **don't touch it, squeeze it, or pick at it.** This might be hard to do—it can be pretty tempting to try to get rid of a pimple. But when you play around with pimples, you can cause even more inflammation by poking at them or opening them up. Plus, the oil from your hands can't help! More important, though, picking at pimples can leave tiny, permanent scars on your face.

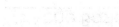

Chapter 8

Treating Acne

Acne is often treated by dermatologists (doctors who specialize in skin problems). These doctors treat all kinds of acne, particularly severe cases. Doctors who are general or family practitioners, pediatricians, or internists may treat patients with milder cases of acne.

The goals of treatment are to heal existing lesions, stop new lesions from forming, prevent scarring, and minimize the psychological stress and embarrassment caused by this disease. Drug treatment is aimed at reducing several problems that play a part in causing acne:

- Abnormal clumping of cells in the follicles

- Increased oil production

- Bacteria

- Inflammation

All medicines can have side effects. Some medicines and side effects are mentioned in this chapter. Some side effects may be more severe than others. You should review the package insert that comes with your medicine and ask your health care provider or pharmacist if you have any questions about the possible side effects.

Depending on the extent of the problem, the doctor may recommend one of several over-the-counter (OTC) medicines and/or prescription medicines. Some of these medicines may be topical (applied to the skin), and others may be oral (taken by mouth).

About This Chapter: Excerpted from "Questions And Answers About Acne," National Institute of Arthritis and Musculoskeletal and Skin Diseases, October 2012.

Treatment For Blackheads, Whiteheads, And Mild Inflammatory Acne

Doctors usually recommend an OTC or prescription topical medicine for people with mild signs of acne. Topical medicine is applied directly to the acne lesions or to the entire area of affected skin.

There are several OTC topical medicines used for mild acne. Each works a little differently. Following are the most common ones:

- **Benzoyl Peroxide:** Destroys *Propionibacterium acnes*, (bacteria that cause acne), and may also reduce oil production

- **Resorcinol:** Can help break down blackheads and whiteheads

- **Salicylic Acid:** Helps break down blackheads and whiteheads. Also helps cut down the shedding of cells lining the hair follicles

- **Sulfur:** Helps break down blackheads and whiteheads

Topical OTC medicines are available in many forms, such as gels, lotions, creams, soaps, or pads. In some people, OTC acne medicines may cause side effects such as skin irritation, burning, or redness, which often get better or go away with continued use of the medicine. If you experience severe or prolonged side effects, you should report them to your doctor.

Treatment For Moderate-To-Severe Inflammatory Acne

People with moderate-to-severe inflammatory acne may be treated with prescription topical or oral medicines, alone or in combination.

Prescription Topical Medicines

Several types of prescription topical medicines are used to treat acne. They include the following:

- **Antibiotics:** Help stop or slow the growth of bacteria and reduce inflammation.

- **Vitamin A Derivatives (Retinoids):** Unplug existing comedones (plural of comedo), allowing other topical medicines, such as antibiotics, to enter the follicles. Some may also help decrease the formation of comedones. These drugs contain an altered form of vitamin A. Some examples are tretinoin, adapalene, and tazarotene.

- **Others:** May destroy *P. acnes* and reduce oil production or help stop or slow the growth of bacteria and reduce inflammation. Some examples are prescription strength benzoyl peroxide, sodium sulfacetamide/sulfur-containing products, or azelaic acid.

Like OTC topical medicines, prescription topical medicines come as creams, lotions, solutions, gels, or pads. Your doctor will consider your skin type when prescribing a product. Creams and lotions provide moisture and tend to be good choices for people with sensitive skin. If you have very oily skin or live in a hot, humid climate, you may prefer an alcohol-based gel or solution, which tends to dry the skin. Your doctor will tell you how to apply the medicine and how often to use it.

For some people, prescription topical medicines cause minor side effects, including stinging, burning, redness, peeling, scaling, or discoloration of the skin. With some medicines, such as tretinoin, these side effects usually decrease or go away after the medicine is used for a period of time. If side effects are severe or don't go away, notify your doctor.

Prescription Oral Medicines

For patients with moderate-to-severe acne, doctors often prescribe oral antibiotics. Oral antibiotics are thought to help control acne by curbing the growth of bacteria and reducing inflammation. Prescription oral and topical medicines may be combined.

Treatment For Severe Nodular Or Cystic Acne

People with nodules or cysts should be treated by a dermatologist. For patients with severe inflammatory acne that does not improve with medicines such as those described above, a doctor may prescribe isotretinoin, a retinoid (vitamin A derivative). It markedly reduces the size of the oil glands so that much less oil is produced. As a result, the growth of bacteria is decreased.

Advantages Of Isotretinoin

Isotretinoin is a very effective medicine that can help prevent scarring. In those patients where acne recurs after a course of isotretinoin, the doctor may institute another course of the same treatment or prescribe other medicines.

41

Disadvantages Of Isotretinoin

Isotretinoin can cause birth defects in the developing fetus of a pregnant woman. **It is important that women of childbearing age are not pregnant and do not get pregnant while taking this medicine.** You should ask your doctor when it is safe to get pregnant after you have stopped taking isotretinoin.

Some people with acne become depressed by the changes in the appearance of their skin. Changes in mood may be intensified during treatment or soon after completing a course of medicines like isotretinoin. There have been a number of reported suicides and suicide attempts in people taking isotretinoin; however, the connection between isotretinoin and suicide or depression is not known. Nevertheless, if you or someone you know feels unusually sad or has other symptoms of depression, such as loss of appetite, loss of interest in once-loved activities, or trouble concentrating, it's important to consult your doctor.

Other possible side effects of isotretinoin include these below:

- Dry eyes, mouth, lips, nose, or skin (very common)

- Itching

- Nosebleeds

- Muscle aches

- Sensitivity to the sun

Treatments For Hormonally Influenced Acne In Women

In some women, acne is caused by an excess of androgen (male) hormones. Clues that this may be the case include hirsutism (excessive growth of hair on the face or body), premenstrual acne flares, irregular menstrual cycles, and elevated blood levels of certain androgens.

The doctor may prescribe one of several drugs to treat women with this type of acne:

- **Birth Control Pills**: Help suppress the androgen produced by the ovaries

- **Low-Dose Corticosteroid Drugs:** Help suppress the androgen produced by the adrenal glands

- **Antiandrogen Drugs:** Reduce the excessive oil production

Side effects of antiandrogen drugs may include irregular menstruation, tender breasts, headaches, and fatigue.

- Poor night vision

- Changes in the blood, such as an increase in fats in the blood (triglycerides and cholesterol)

- Change in liver function

To be able to determine if isotretinoin should be stopped if side effects occur, your doctor may test your blood before you start treatment and periodically during treatment.

Other Treatments For Acne

Doctors may use other types of procedures in addition to drug therapy to treat patients with acne. For example, the doctor may remove the patient's comedones during office visits. Sometimes the doctor will inject corticosteroids directly into lesions to help reduce the size and pain of inflamed cysts and nodules.

Early treatment is the best way to prevent acne scars. Once scarring has occurred, the doctor may suggest a medical or surgical procedure to help reduce the scars. A superficial laser may be used to treat irregular scars. Dermabrasion (or microdermabrasion), which is a form of "sanding down" scars, is sometimes used. Another treatment option for deep scars caused by cystic acne is the transfer of fat from another part of the body to the scar. A doctor may also inject a synthetic filling material under the scar to improve its appearance.

Chapter 9

Isotretinoin Warning

Isotretinoin

- **Pronunciation:** eye soe tret' i noyn
- **Brand Names:** Absorica , Accutane, Amnesteem , Claravis , Myorisan, Sotret

Important Warning

For All Patients

Isotretinoin must not be taken by patients who are pregnant or who may become pregnant. There is a high risk that isotretinoin will cause loss of the pregnancy, or will cause the baby to be born too early, to die shortly after birth, or to be born with birth defects (physical problems that are present at birth).

A program called iPLEDGE has been set up to make sure that pregnant women do not take isotretinoin and that women do not become pregnant while taking isotretinoin. All patients, including women who cannot become pregnant and men, can get isotretinoin only if they are registered with iPLEDGE, have a prescription from a doctor who is registered with iPLEDGE, and fill the prescription at a pharmacy that is registered with iPLEDGE. Do not buy isotretinoin over the internet.

You will receive information about the risks of taking isotretinoin and must sign an informed consent sheet stating that you understand this information before you can receive the medication. You will need to see your doctor every month during your treatment to talk about your condition and the side effects you are experiencing. At each visit, your doctor may give you a prescription for up to a 30-day supply of medication with no refills. If you are a woman who can become pregnant, you will also need to have a pregnancy test in an approved lab each month and have your prescription filled and picked up within seven days of your pregnancy test. If you are a man or if you are a woman who cannot become pregnant, you must have this prescription filled and picked up within 30 days of your doctor visit. Your pharmacist cannot dispense your medication if you come to pick it up after the allowed time period has passed.

Tell your doctor if you do not understand everything you were told about isotretinoin and the iPLEDGE program or if you do not think you will be able to keep appointments or fill your prescription on schedule every month.

Your doctor will give you an identification number and card when you start your treatment. You will need this number to fill your prescriptions and to get information from the iPLEDGE website and phone line. Keep the card in a safe place where it will not get lost. If you do lose your card, you can ask for a replacement through the website or phone line.

Do not donate blood while you are taking isotretinoin and for one month after your treatment.

Do not share isotretinoin with anyone else, even someone who has the same symptoms that you have. Your doctor or pharmacist will give you the manufacturer's patient information sheet (Medication Guide) when you begin treatment with isotretinoin and each time you refill your prescription. Read the information carefully and ask your doctor or pharmacist if you have any questions. You can also visit the Food and Drug Administration (FDA) website (http://www.fda.gov/Drugs), the manufacturer's website, or the iPLEDGE program website (http://www.ipledgeprogram.com) to obtain the Medication Guide.

Talk to your doctor about the risks of taking isotretinoin.

For Female Patients

If you can become pregnant, you will need to meet certain requirements during your treatment with isotretinoin. You need to meet these requirements even if you have not started menstruating (having monthly periods) or have had a tubal ligation ('tubes tied'; surgery to prevent pregnancy). You may be excused from meeting these requirements only if you have not menstruated for 12 months in a row and your doctor says you have passed menopause (change of life) or you have had surgery to remove your uterus and/or both ovaries. If none of these are true for you, then you must meet the requirements below.

You must use two acceptable forms of birth control for one month before you begin to take isotretinoin, during your treatment and for one month after your treatment. Your doctor will tell you which forms of birth control are acceptable and will give you written information about birth control. You can also have a free visit with a doctor or family planning expert to talk about birth control that is right for you. You must use these two forms of birth control at all times unless you can promise that you will not have any sexual contact with a male for one month before your treatment, during your treatment, and for one month after your treatment.

If you choose to take isotretinoin, it is your responsibility to avoid pregnancy for one month before, during, and for one month after your treatment. You must understand that any form of birth control can fail. Therefore, it is very important to decrease the risk of accidental pregnancy by using two forms of birth control at all times. Tell your doctor if you do not understand everything you were told about birth control or you do not think that you will be able to use two forms of birth control at all times. If you plan to use oral contraceptives (birth control pills) while taking isotretinoin, tell your doctor the name of the pill you will use. Isotretinoin interferes with the action of micro-dosed progestin ('minipill') oral contraceptives (Ovrette, Micronor, Nor-QD). Do not use this type of birth control while taking isotretinoin.

If you plan to use hormonal contraceptives (birth control pills, patches, implants, injections, rings, or intrauterine devices), be sure to tell your doctor about all the medications, vitamins, and herbal supplements you are taking. Many medications interfere with the action of hormonal contraceptives. Do not take St. John's wort if you are using any type of hormonal contraceptive.

You must have two negative pregnancy tests before you can begin to take isotretinoin. Your doctor will tell you when and where to have these tests. You will also need to be tested for pregnancy in a laboratory each month during your treatment, when you take your last dose and 30 days after you take your last dose.

You will need to contact the iPLEDGE system by phone or the internet every month to confirm the two forms of birth control you are using and to answer two questions about the iPLEDGE program. You will only be able to continue to get isotretinoin if you have done this, if you have visited your doctor to talk about how you are feeling and how you are using your birth control and if you have had a negative pregnancy test within the past seven days.

Stop taking isotretinoin and call your doctor right away if you think you are pregnant, you miss a menstrual period, or you have sex without using two forms of birth control. If you become pregnant during your treatment or within 30 days after your treatment, your doctor will contact the iPLEDGE program, the manufacturer of isotretinoin, and the Food and Drug

Administration (FDA). You will also talk with a doctor who specializes in problems during pregnancy who can help you make choices that are best for you and your baby. Information about your health and your baby's health will be used to help doctors learn more about the effects of isotretinoin on unborn babies.

For Male Patients

A very small amount of isotretinoin will probably be present in your semen when you take prescribed doses of this medication. It is not known if this small amount of isotretinoin may harm the fetus if your partner is or becomes pregnant. Tell your doctor if your partner is pregnant, plans to become pregnant, or becomes pregnant during your treatment with isotretinoin.

Questions About Isotretinoin

Why is this medicine prescribed?

Isotretinoin is used to treat severe recalcitrant nodular acne (a certain type of severe acne) that has not been helped by other treatments, such as antibiotics. Isotretinoin is in a class of medications called retinoids. It works by slowing the production of certain natural substances that can cause acne.

How should this medicine be used?

Isotretinoin comes as a capsule to take by mouth. Isotretinoin is usually taken twice a day with meals for four to five months at a time. Follow the directions on your prescription label carefully, and ask your doctor or pharmacist to explain any part you do not understand.

Take isotretinoin exactly as directed. Do not take more or less of it or take it more often than prescribed by your doctor.

Swallow the capsules whole with a full glass of liquid. Do not chew or suck on the capsules.

Your doctor will probably start you on an average dose of isotretinoin and increase or decrease your dose depending on how well you respond to the medication and the side effects you experience. Follow these directions carefully and ask your doctor or pharmacist if you are not sure how much isotretinoin you should take.

It may take several weeks or longer for you to feel the full benefit of isotretinoin. Your acne may get worse during the beginning of your treatment with isotretinoin. This is normal and does not mean that the medication is not working. Your acne may continue to improve even after you finish your treatment with isotretinoin.

Are there other uses for this medication?

Isotretinoin has been used to treat certain other skin conditions and some types of cancer. Talk to your doctor about the possible risks of using this medication for your condition.

This medication may be prescribed for other uses. Ask your doctor or pharmacist for more information.

What special precautions should I follow?

Before taking isotretinoin:

- Tell your doctor and pharmacist if you are allergic to isotretinoin, vitamin A, any other medications, or any of the ingredients in isotretinoin capsules. Ask your pharmacist or check the Medication Guide for a list of the inactive ingredients.

- Tell your doctor and pharmacist what prescription and nonprescription medications, vitamins, herbal products, and nutritional supplements you are taking or plan to take. Be sure to mention medications for seizures such as phenytoin (Dilantin); medications for mental illness; oral steroids such as dexamethasone (Decadron, Dexone), methylprednisolone (Medrol), and prednisone (Deltasone); tetracycline antibiotics such as demeclocycline (Declomycin), doxycycline (Monodox, Vibramycin, others), minocycline (Minocin, Vectrin), oxytetracycline (Terramycin), and tetracycline (Sumycin, Tetrex, others); and vitamin A supplements. Your doctor may need to change the doses of your medications or monitor you carefully for side effects.

- Tell your doctor if you or anyone in your family has thought about or attempted suicide and if you or anyone in your family has or has ever had depression, mental illness, diabetes, asthma, osteoporosis (a condition in which the bones are fragile and break easily), osteomalacia (weak bones due to a lack of vitamin D or difficulty absorbing this vitamin), or other conditions that cause weak bones, a high triglyceride (fats in the blood) level, a lipid metabolism disorder (any condition that makes it difficult for your body to process fats), anorexia nervosa (an eating disorder in which very little is eaten), or heart or liver disease. Also tell your doctor if you are overweight or if you drink or have ever drunk large amounts of alcohol.

- Do not breast-feed while you are taking isotretinoin and for one month after you stop taking isotretinoin.

- Plan to avoid unnecessary or prolonged exposure to sunlight and to wear protective clothing, sunglasses, and sunscreen. Isotretinoin may make your skin sensitive to sunlight.

- You should know that isotretinoin may cause changes in your thoughts, behavior, or mental health. Some patients who took isotretinoin have developed depression or psychosis (loss of contact with reality), have become violent, have thought about killing or hurting themselves, and have tried or succeeded in doing so. You or your family should call your doctor right away if you experience any of the following symptoms: anxiety, sadness, crying spells, loss of interest in activities you used to enjoy, poor performance at school or work, sleeping more than usual, difficulty falling asleep or staying asleep, irritability, anger, aggression, changes in appetite or weight, difficulty concentrating, withdrawing from friends or family, lack of energy, feelings of worthlessness or guilt, thinking about killing or hurting yourself, acting on dangerous thoughts, or hallucinations (seeing or hearing things that do not exist). Be sure that your family members know which symptoms are serious so that they can call the doctor if you are unable to seek treatment on your own.

- You should know that isotretinoin may cause your eyes to feel dry and make wearing contact lenses uncomfortable during and after your treatment.

- You should know that isotretinoin may limit your ability to see in the dark. This problem may begin suddenly at any time during your treatment and may continue after your treatment is stopped. Be very careful when you drive or operate machinery at night.

- Plan to avoid hair removal by waxing, laser skin treatments, and dermabrasion (surgical smoothing of the skin) while you are taking isotretinoin and for six months after your treatment. Isotretinoin increases the risk that you will develop scars from these treatments. Ask your doctor when you can safely undergo these treatments.

- Talk to your doctor before you participate in hard physical activity such as sports. Isotretinoin may cause the bones to weaken or thicken abnormally and may increase the risk of certain bone injuries in people who perform some types of physical activity. If you break a bone during your treatment, be sure to tell all your healthcare providers that you are taking isotretinoin.

What special dietary instructions should I follow?

Unless your doctor tells you otherwise, continue your normal diet.

What should I do if I forget to take a dose?

Skip the missed dose and continue your regular dosing schedule. Do not take a double dose to make up for a missed one.

What side effects can this medicine cause?

Isotretinoin may cause side effects. Tell your doctor if any of these symptoms are severe or do not go away:

- Red, cracked, and sore lips
- Dry skin, eyes, mouth, or nose
- Nosebleeds
- Changes in skin color
- Peeling skin on the palms of the hands and soles of the feet
- Changes in the nails
- Slowed healing of cuts or sores
- Bleeding or swollen gums
- Hair loss or unwanted hair growth
- Sweating
- Flushing
- Voice changes
- Tiredness
- Cold symptoms

Some side effects can be serious. If you experience any of the following symptoms or those listed in the IMPORTANT WARNING or SPECIAL PRECAUTIONS sections, stop taking isotretinoin and call your doctor or get emergency medical treatment immediately:

- Headache
- Blurred vision
- Dizziness
- Nausea
- Vomiting
- Seizures
- Slow or difficult speech
- Weakness or numbness of one part or side of the body

- Stomach pain
- Chest pain
- Difficulty swallowing or pain when swallowing
- New or worsening heartburn
- Diarrhea
- Rectal bleeding
- Yellowing of the skin or eyes
- Dark colored urine
- Back, bone, joint, or muscle pain
- Muscle weakness
- Difficulty hearing
- Ringing in the ears
- Vision problems
- Painful or constant dryness of the eyes
- Unusual thirst
- Frequent urination
- Trouble breathing
- Fainting
- Fast or pounding heartbeat
- Red, swollen, itchy, or teary eyes
- Fever
- Rash
- Peeling or blistering skin, especially on the legs, arms, or face
- Sores in the mouth, throat, nose, or eyes
- Red patches or bruises on the legs
- Swelling of the eyes, face, lips, tongue, throat, arms, hands, feet, ankles, or lower legs
- Difficulty swallowing or pain when swallowing

Isotretinoin may cause the bones to stop growing too soon in teenagers. Talk to your child's* doctor about the risks of giving this medication to your child.*

Isotretinoin may cause other side effects. Call your doctor if you have any unusual problems while taking this medication.

If you experience a serious side effect, you or your doctor may send a report to the Food and Drug Administration's (FDA) MedWatch Adverse Event Reporting program online [at http://www.fda.gov/Safety/MedWatch] or by phone [1-800-332-1088].

What should I know about storage and disposal of this medication?

Keep this medication in the container it came in, tightly closed, and out of reach of children. Store it at room temperature and away from excess heat and moisture (not in the bathroom). Throw away any medication that is outdated or no longer needed. Talk to your pharmacist about the proper disposal of your medication.

What should I do in case of overdose?

In case of overdose, call your local poison control center at 1-800-222-1222. If the victim has collapsed or is not breathing, call local emergency services at 911.

Symptoms of overdose may include the following:

- Vomiting
- Flushing
- Severe chapped lips
- Stomach pain
- Headache
- Dizziness
- Loss of coordination

Anyone who has taken an overdose of isotretinoin should know about the risk of birth defects caused by isotretinoin and should not donate blood for one month after the overdose. Pregnant woman should talk to their doctors about the risks of continuing the pregnancy after the overdose. Women who can become pregnant should use two forms of birth control for one month after the overdose. Men whose partners are or may become pregnant should use condoms or avoid sexual contact with that partner for one month after the overdose because isotretinoin may be present in the semen.

What other information should I know?

Keep all appointments with your doctor and the laboratory. Your doctor will order certain lab tests to check your response to isotretinoin.

This chapter does not contain all the possible information about this drug. Your doctor or pharmacist can give you additional information to answer any questions you may have.

*Note

Although some of the text in this chapter addresses parents, the information is still pertinent to teens.

Chapter 10

Differences Between Boys And Girls In Their Experiences With Acne

Acne Tips For Boys

Acne is a skin condition that occurs because of clogged pores that result from an over-production of sebum. (Sebum is an oily substance secreted by the sebaceous glands under the skin of the face, neck, shoulders, back, and chest.)

How is acne different in boys and young men?

Acne starts to appear during adolescence because the rising hormone levels during puberty trigger higher levels of sebum production. Puberty starts later in boys than in girls, so boys tend to get acne at a later age than girls.

Boys also develop higher levels of androgens, a type of hormone associated with male traits, such as a greater muscle mass, deeper voice, and body hair. These androgens also stimulate the sebaceous glands, and can lead to more severe cases of acne in boys.

Boys are more likely to get acne on the chest and back, and their acne tends to be more severe and long lasting.

Boys who shave may also be at a higher risk for acne flares, especially if using dull, low-quality razors or not using shaving cream.

Finally, boys tend to be less likely to use acne skin care products than girls, so they may not be aware of the topical treatments available for acne. They may also be less likely to seek help for their acne.

About This Chapter: "Acne Tips for Boys," and "Acne Tips for Girls," by Mark Becker, M.D., reprinted with permission from http://fromyourdoctor.com. © 2012 Vivacare, Inc. All rights reserved.

What acne treatments are available for boys and young men?

Acne treatments for boys and girls are very similar. The goal of acne treatment is to kill the bacteria that causes acne lesions to become inflamed (*P. acnes*), remove dead skin cells, and lower sebum production.

Many cases of mild acne can be treated with over-the-counter medications (benzoyl peroxide), but your dermatologist may recommend something stronger to avoid prolonging the acne since persistent acne increases the risk of developing acne scars. In that case, you may be prescribed a topical or oral antibiotic, a prescription-strength topical retinoid, or both.

Topical retinoids are the mainstay of acne therapy. Medications in this class include generic tretinoin, Differin (adapalene), Tazorac (tazarotene), Retin-A Micro (tretinoin), and newer combination therapies, such as Epiduo (adapalene plus benzoyl peroxide), and Ziana (tretinoin plus clindamycin).

The worst cases of acne may require the use of isotretinoin (formerly referred to as Accutane). Isotretinoin is a very effective oral medication for acne that carries potentially serious side effects. Patients taking isotretinoin are required to participate in the iPledge program that helps to monitor for side effects.

Your doctor will recommend an acne treatment plan based on several factors, including:

- The severity of the acne
- The presence of acne scars
- The response to past acne treatments
- Other medical conditions

Stick to your acne treatment plan.

No acne medication can do its job properly unless it is given time to work. **You must be patient.**

It's very important take your acne medication as directed, for as long as directed. If you don't see results right away, don't be discouraged. Your medication is hard at work preventing new lesions from forming. Stopping treatment early will likely cause pimples and zits to reappear.

What can boys and young men do to prevent acne?

- Cleanse your skin twice a day with a mild soap; avoid scrubbing hard with a washcloth—it won't help the acne go away and it may worsen the condition by irritating the skin.

- Teens tend to get acne in the T-zone of the face (chin, nose, and forehead), so use an oil-free moisturizer if possible, and use less moisturizer in those areas.

- If your hair is long enough to touch your face, wash it daily to keep oil away from your skin. Avoid letting hair products touch your face.

- Wash your face gently after working around oily substances (such as in a hot kitchen or gas station).

- Bathe or wash your face after exercising, especially areas of the body that come into close, prolonged contact with sports gear (such as helmets, shoulder pads, backpacks, or bike shorts).

- Don't touch your face, because the oil and bacteria from your hands can worsen your acne.

- Avoid the temptation to pick at or squeeze your pimples or zits—this can irritate them and cause scarring.

- **When using a medication,** give it time to work. Your skin may look worse before it looks better, and it may be six to eight weeks before you see improvement. If you don't see results after two months, talk to your dermatologist about switching treatments or adjusting your dosage.

- The sooner you treat your acne, the easier it will be to bring it under control. Virtually any case of acne is treatable, and it's much easier to eliminate lesions in the early stages, which keeps them from growing and prevents scarring.

Acne Tips For Girls

Acne is a skin condition that occurs because of clogged pores that result from an over-production of sebum. (Sebum is an oily substance secreted by the sebaceous glands under the skin of the face, neck, shoulders, back, and chest.)

How is acne different in girls and young women?

Acne lesions first start to appear during puberty as hormone levels rise. Puberty typically starts at a younger age in girls than boys, so girls often start to develop acne at a younger age than boys.

In addition to the puberty-related changes experienced by all teens, girls must also contend with the hormonal swings of menstruation, so acne may flare at certain times during the menstrual cycle.

Girls also differ in their response to acne. Because they are more likely to use acne skin care products than boys, they are often more receptive to using various over-the-counter acne treatments that can offer relief for mild cases of acne.

What acne treatments are available for girls and young women?

The goal of acne treatment is to kill bacteria, remove dead skin cells, and lower sebum production. The dermatologist will choose a treatment based on the severity of the acne, which could be mild, moderate, or severe.

Many mild cases may respond to the use of over-the-counter medications, but sometimes your physician will recommend something stronger to avoid prolonging the acne and the risk of scarring. In that case, you may be prescribed a topical or oral antibiotic, a prescription-strength topical retinoid, or both.

Topical retinoids are the mainstay of acne therapy. Medications in this class include generic tretinoin, Differin (adapalene), Tazorac (tazarotene), Retin-A Micro (tretinoin), and newer combination therapies, such as Epiduo (adapalene plus benzoyl peroxide), and Ziana (tretinoin plus clindamycin).

The worst cases of acne may require the use of isotretinoin (formerly referred to as Accutane). Isotretinoin is a very effective oral medication for acne that carries potentially serious side effects. Patients taking isotretinoin are required to participate in the iPledge program that helps to monitor for side effects.

Your doctor will recommend an acne treatment plan based on several factors, including:

• The severity of the acne
• The presence of acne scars
• The response to past acne treatments
• Other medical conditions

Stick with your acne treatment plan.

No acne medication can do its job properly unless it is given time to work. It's very important to be patient and take your medication as directed, for as long as directed. If you don't see results right away, don't be discouraged.

Your acne medication is hard at work preventing new lesions from forming. Stopping acne treatment early will likely cause pimples and zits to reappear.

What should you know about skincare products and acne?

In choosing cosmetics and skin cleansers, girls have many acne-fighting products to choose from. To kill *P. acnes* and other acne-causing bacteria, find a gentle cleanser containing benzoyl peroxide, sulfur, or salicylic acid.

When shopping for makeup, hair products, moisturizers, and other cosmetics, avoid heavy, greasy formulations that could clog pores and worsen your acne. Choose products labeled noncomedogenic or non-acnegenic, as these are less likely to block your pores. Today, you can even find acne-medicated makeup and spot treatments, which conceal and heal your lesions at the same time.

Chapter 11

Polycystic Ovarian Syndrome And Acne

What is PCOS?

Polycystic (say: pah-lee-SIS-tik) ovary syndrome (PCOS) is a common hormone imbalance that affects around one out of ten women. Girls as young as 11 can get PCOS. This chapter is for you if you have PCOS or are struggling with common signs of the condition, such as irregular periods, acne, or unwanted body hair. Read answers to commonly asked questions about PCOS below.

What are the signs of PCOS?

These are some common signs of PCOS:

- Irregular periods or none at all

- Pelvic pain

- Extra hair on your face or other parts of your body, called "hirsutism" (say: HER-soo-tism)

- Acne

- Weight gain and/or trouble losing weight

- Patches of dark skin on the back of your neck and other areas

If you have some or all of the above signs, you might have PCOS. There may be other reasons that you might have one or more of these signs. Only your doctor can tell for sure.

About This Chapter: From "What Is PCOS?" Office on Women's Health (girlshealth.gov), October 13, 2010.

What causes PCOS?

No one knows the exact cause of PCOS. We do know that it comes from problems with hormones, or natural body chemicals. Many girls with PCOS have too much insulin, a hormone that helps turn food into energy. Extra insulin can cause the darkened skin you may have on your neck, behind your knees, and other places. Also, having too much insulin may cause your body to make more of hormones called androgens (say: AN-druh-junz). Although these hormones cause male traits, females have them too. It's the extra androgen that can lead to acne, excess body hair, weight gain, and irregular periods.

What tests are used to diagnose PCOS?

If you think you may have PCOS, it's smart to see your doctor. And knowing what to expect during the appointment can make it less stressful. Here's a list of some of what you might experience:

- Questions from your doctor about your menstrual cycle and your health.

- A physical examination, including a measure of your body mass index (BMI) and waist size. You may also have an examination of the outside of your vagina.

- A blood test to check your hormone levels and blood sugar levels.

Does PCOS mean I have cysts on my ovaries?

The term "polycystic ovaries" means that there are lots of tiny cysts, or bumps, inside of the ovaries. Some young women with PCOS have these cysts; many others do not. Even if you do have them, they are not harmful and do not need to be removed.

Will PCOS affect my ability to have children some day?

Women with PCOS may have trouble getting pregnant, but some women have no trouble at all. If you are concerned about your fertility (ability to get pregnant) in the future, talk to your doctor about all the new options available. These include medications to lower your insulin levels and to help you ovulate—or release an egg—each month.

Does PCOS put me at risk for other conditions?

If you have PCOS, you may be at higher risk for other health problems. These are some possible conditions:

- Diabetes

- High cholesterol

- High blood pressure

- Heart disease

Women with PCOS often have low levels of the hormone progesterone. Progesterone causes the endometrium to shed each month as your period. If you don't have enough progesterone, the endometrium becomes thick, which can cause heavy or irregular bleeding. In time, this can lead to endometrial hyperplasia, which means the uterus gets thick with abnormal cells, or cancer.

Getting your PCOS symptoms under control at an early age may help to reduce these risks.

What is the treatment for PCOS?

There is no cure for PCOS, but there are lots of ways to treat it. You may use a few of them or different ones at different times, depending on your symptoms.

One great way to deal with PCOS is to eat well and exercise. If you are overweight, losing weight may help with symptoms and may reduce health risks related to PCOS. Don't smoke—or try to quit if you've started.

Birth control pills are a very common form of treatment for PCOS. Birth control pills contain hormones that can help in several ways:

- Correct the PCOS hormone imbalance

- Lower the level of male hormones, which will lessen acne and hair growth

- Regulate your menstrual period

- Lower the risk of endometrial cancer (which is higher in young women who don't ovulate regularly)

Metformin is another medicine that may help with ovulation and other PCOS issues. Your doctor may also ask you to take a blood test to measure your body's ability to use glucose. (Glucose is a kind of sugar that your body breaks food into to use for fuel.) This test will help find out if you are more likely to get diabetes, which sometimes is also treated with metformin.

Antiandrogens work to reduce the effects of the male hormones on girls with PCOS. They can help clear up acne and hair growth. You can also deal with unwanted hair through electrolysis, hair removal creams, and laser treatment. There are lots of other options for treating acne.

What if I have worries about having PCOS?

If you have been told you have PCOS, you may feel frustrated or sad. You may also feel relieved that at last there is an explanation for the problems you have been having with keeping a healthy weight, having excess body hair, acne, or irregular periods. At the same time, having a diagnosis without an easy cure can be difficult. Keep in mind that there are treatments for many of the problems that PCOS can cause. And it is important for girls with PCOS to know they are not alone. Finding a doctor who knows a lot about PCOS and who you feel comfortable talking to is very important. Keeping a positive attitude and working on a healthy lifestyle even when results seem to take a long time is very important too! Many girls with PCOS tell us that talking with a counselor about their concerns can be very helpful. Other girls recommend internet chats.

> Having a healthy lifestyle through ups and downs is the first step to living with PCOS!

Chapter 12

Psychological Effects Of Acne

Acne can have profound social and psychological effects. These are not necessarily related to its clinical severity. Even mild acne can be significantly disabling. Acne can affect people of all ages but it predominantly occurs during the teenage years; approximately 85 percent of people between the ages of 12 and 25 develop acne.

What Problems Does It Cause?

The psychological and social impacts of acne are a huge concern especially because it affects adolescents at a time they are developing their personalities. During this time, peer acceptance is very important to the teenager and unfortunately it has been found that physical appearance and attractiveness is highly linked with peer status.

In recent years, open discussions between patients and medical professionals have revealed the impact acne has on one's psyche. The following are some of the problems that patients with acne may face:

Self-Esteem And Body Image

- Some embarrassed acne patients avoid eye contact.

- Some acne sufferers grow their hair long to cover the face. Girls tend to wear heavy make-up to disguise the pimples, even though they know this sometimes aggravates the condition. Boys often comment, "Acne is not such a problem for girls because they can wear make-up."

- Truncal acne can reduce participation in sport such as swimming or rugby because of the need to disrobe in public changing rooms.

Social Withdrawal/Relationship Building

- Acne, especially when it affects the face, provokes cruel taunts from other teenagers.

- Some find it hard to form new relationships, especially with the opposite sex.

- At a time when teenagers are learning to form relationships, those with acne may lack the self-confidence to go out and make these bonds. They become shy and even reclusive. The main concern is a fear of negative appraisal by others. In extreme cases a social phobia can develop.

Education/Work

- Some refuse to go school leading to poor academic performance and possibly future unemployment.

- Some take sick days from work, risking their jobs or livelihood.

- Acne may reduce career choices, ruling out occupations such as modeling that depend upon personal appearance.

- Acne patients are less successful in job applications; their lack of confidence being as important as the potential employers' reaction to their spotty skin.

- More people who have acne are unemployed than people who do not have acne are.

- Many young adults with acne seek medical help as they enter the workforce, where they perceive that acne is unacceptable and that they "should have grown out of it by now."

Acne And Depression

In some patients the distress of acne may result in depression. This must be recognized and managed.

Signs of depression include:

- Loss of appetite

- Lethargy

- Mood disturbance

- Behavioral problems
- Wakefulness
- Spontaneous crying
- Feelings of unworthiness

In teenagers depression may manifest as social withdrawal (retreat to the bedroom or avoidance of peers) or impaired school performance (lower grades or missed assignments). Worse still, severe depression from acne has resulted in attempted suicide and, unfortunately, successful suicide. Worrying statements include "I don't want to wake up in the morning," "I'd be better off dead," "I'm worthless," "You'd be better off without me." Parents, friends, and school counselors need to take heed when they start to hear these types of comments.

Rarely, depression can be associated with acne treatment, particularly isotretinoin. There is considerable doubt that the drug has caused the problem and it seems much more likely that it results from the acne and psychological disturbances described above.

Regardless of the cause, depression must be recognized and managed early. If you think you may be depressed, contact your dermatologist or family doctor urgently for advice.

Dysmorphophobic Acne

Some patients with only minor acne suffer from disturbed body image. Even in the absence of lesions, they consider they have severe acne and may suffer many of the psychological and social symptoms described above. They are said to have "dysmorphophobic acne." If this is their only abnormal behavioral symptom, they respond well to oral isotretinoin therapy. A low dose of this may be required long term as even slight recurrence of oily skin may unduly concern the patient. Some severe cases of dysmorphophobia have a more global mental disorder similar to anorexia nervosa. They require expert dermatological and psychiatric assistance.

Seeking Help

If your acne is interfering significantly with your life, particularly if it is resulting in any of the problems described above, seek help promptly from your family physician or dermatologist.

Tell your doctor all your concerns so that he or she will take your acne seriously. Most cases of acne can be controlled and sometimes cured with treatment, using one or more of the following preparations:

- Over-the-counter topical acne creams, lotions, or gels for mild cases

- Prescription medications, both topical and oral, that are available only through a physician

Depression is an illness that can nearly always be treated effectively. See your family doctor for advice and if necessary referral to a health professional specializing in mental illness.

Suitable treatments may include:

- Antidepressant medication

- Psychological treatments to overcome the negative thinking, anxiety, and avoidance that often accompany depression

- Counseling to help build confidence and rebuild self-esteem

- Group therapy

It is important that a teenager's anxiety over their acne is managed appropriately.

Part Three
Infectious Conditions Of The Skin

Chapter 13

Bacterial Infections: Cellulitis, Impetigo, Boils, And Necrotizing Fasciitis

Bacterial Skin Infections

Bacteria such as some *Staphylococcus* species, *Corynebacterium* spp., *Brevibacterium* spp., and *Acinetobacter* live on normal skin and cause no harm. Propionibacteria live in the hair follicles of adult skin and contribute to acne.

Some bacteria invade normal skin, broken skin from eczema/dermatitis, or wounds (causing wound infection). Bacteria, like viruses, may also sometimes result in exanthems (rashes). The most common bacteria to cause skin infections are:

- *Staphylococcus aureus*

  - Folliculitis

  - Furunculosis (boils)

  - Impetigo (school sores)

  - Methicillin (meticillin) resistant *Staph. aureus*

  - Staphylococcal scalded skin syndrome

  - Toxic shock syndrome

  - Tropical pyomyositis

  - Botryomycosis (pyoderma vegetans)

- *Streptococcus pyogenes*
  - Cellulitis
  - Erysipelas
  - Impetigo
  - Necrotizing fasciitis
  - Scarlet fever
  - Rheumatic fever, erythema marginatum
- Overgrowth of *Corynebacterium* spp. (erythrisma, pitted keratolysis, and trichomycosis axillaris)

Boils

Boils (also called furuncles) are a deep infection of hair follicles.

What Are Boils?

Boils present as one or more tender red spots, lumps, or pustules. Careful inspection reveals that the boil is centered on a hair follicle. A boil is a deep form of bacterial folliculitis; superficial folliculitis is sometimes present at the same time. *Staphylococcus aureus* can be cultured from the skin lesions.

If there are multiple heads, the lesion is called a "carbuncle." Large boils form abscesses, defined as an accumulation of pus within a cavity. Cellulitis may also occur, i.e., infection of the surrounding tissues, and this may cause fever and illness.

Why Do Boils Occur?

Most people with boils are otherwise healthy and have good personal hygiene. They do however carry *Staph. aureus* on the surface of their skins (*Staph.* carrier state). Why this occurs is usually not known, but it is estimated that 10–20 percent of the population are *Staph.* carriers.

Staph. aureus is most commonly carried in the nostrils, armpits, between the legs, and in the cleft between the buttocks. It may be transferred to other sites from the nostrils via the fingernails.

Tiny nicks or grazes or something rubbing against the skin can inoculate the *Staph.* germ into the wall of a hair follicle which is a 'weak point' in the skin's defenses. Once inoculated, the bacteria cause a boil which goes on to run its usual course of about 10 days.

Although most people with boils are otherwise healthy, boils are sometimes related to immune deficiency, anemia, diabetes, or iron deficiency.

Treatment

General measures:

- Consult your doctor about your general health.

- If you are overweight, try to reduce your weight; take regular exercise.

- Follow a balanced healthy diet with meat, plenty of fruit and vegetables.

- Wash your whole body once a day with soap or cleanser and water. Wash your hands several times daily or use antiseptic hand rubs.

- Don't share your washcloth or towel with other family members.

- Maintain a clean handkerchief and don't pick your nose.

- Change your underclothes and night attire regularly.

- Consider modifying leisure activities that cause sweating and friction from clothing, such as squash and jogging.

- If you are iron deficient, a course of iron tablets may help reduce infection.

- 1,000 mg of vitamin C each day has also been advocated to improve deficient neutrophil function.

Skin cleansing regime—ask your doctor for specific advice. Some suggestions:

- Antiseptic or antibacterial soap in your daily bath or shower for a week then twice weekly for several weeks. The cleanser may cause a little dryness.

- Use a hand sanitizer regularly to reduce the chance of re-infecting yourself or others with contaminated hands.

- Antiseptic or antibiotic ointment or gel to apply to the inside of the nostrils.

- Wipe the entire skin surface daily for a week with 70% isopropyl alcohol in water (this will make the skin dry).

- Apply a topical antiseptic such as povidone iodine or chlorhexidine cream to the boils and cover with a square of gauze.

- Your doctor may prescribe an oral antibiotic (usually the penicillin antibiotic flucloxacillin), sometimes for several weeks.

- Other members of the family with boils should also follow a skin cleansing regime. Your doctor may also advise the family to apply topical antibiotic to their nostrils in case they are *Staph. aureus* carriers as well.

- If the boils fail to clear up, a swab should be taken for microbiological culture, in case of methicillin (meticillin) resistant staphylococci.

- Sometimes, special antibiotics may be prescribed on the recommendation of a specialist, including fusidic acid, clindamycin, rifampicin, and cephalosporins.

Cellulitis

Cellulitis is a common bacterial infection of the skin, which can affect all ages. It usually affects a limb but can occur anywhere on the body. Symptoms and signs are usually localized to the affected area but patients can become generally unwell with fevers, chills and shakes (bacteremia).

Severe or rapidly progressive cellulitis may lead to septicemia (blood poisoning), necrotizing fasciitis (a more serious soft tissue infection), or endocarditis (heart valve infection).

Predisposing Factors

Cellulitis is more common in some situations:

- Previous episode(s) of cellulitis
- Venous disease (e.g., gravitational eczema, leg ulceration) and/or lymphedema
- Current or prior injury (e.g., trauma, surgical wounds, radiotherapy)
- Diabetes
- Alcoholism
- Obesity
- Pregnancy
- *Tinea pedis* (or athlete's foot) in the toes of the affected limb

Clinical Features

Some or all of the following features may be seen over the affected skin:

- Redness
- Swelling

- Increased warmth

- Tenderness

- Blistering

- Abscess

- Erosions and ulceration

If there is no increased warmth over the skin it is unlikely to be cellulitis.

Lymphangitis is a red line originating from the cellulitis and leading to tender swollen lymph glands draining the affected area (e.g., in the groin with a leg cellulitis). It is caused by infection within the lymph vessels.

After successful treatment, the skin may flake or peel off as it heals.

What May Cause Cellulitis?

Cellulitis is caused by bacterial infection. It can occur by itself, or complicate an underlying skin condition or wound. The most common infecting organisms are *Streptococcus pyogenes* (two-thirds of cases) and *Staphylococcus aureus* (one-third). Rare causes of cellulitis include:

- *Pseudomonas aeruginosa*, particularly following a puncture wound involving the foot or hand

- *Haemophilus influenzae* in children with facial cellulitis

- Anaerobes, *Eikenella, Streptococcus viridans* from human bites

- *Pasteurella multocida* from cat or dog bites

- *Vibrio vulnificus* from salt water exposure; e.g., following coral injury

- *Aeromonas* from fresh water exposure; e.g., following leech bites

- *Erysipelothrix* (erysipeloid) affecting a butcher

How Is The Diagnosis Made?

The diagnosis of cellulitis is based on the clinical features. If any pustules, crusts, or erosions are present, a swab should be taken for culture. A complete blood count is likely to show leukocytosis (raised white cell count). Blood cultures may be of use if a patient has a high fever or is otherwise very unwell.

Occasionally further investigations are required to rule out other possible diagnoses such as deep vein thrombosis of the leg, radiation damage following radiotherapy, or inflammatory breast cancer.

Treatment

Cellulitis is potentially serious and should be assessed by a medical practitioner promptly.

Most patients can be treated with oral antibiotics at home, usually for 5 to 10 days. However if there are signs of systemic illness or extensive cellulitis, treatment may require intravenous antibiotics either as an outpatient or in hospital. Treatment for uncomplicated cellulitis is usually for 10 to 14 days but antibiotics should be continued until all signs of infection have cleared (redness, pain and, swelling)—sometimes for several months.

Oral antibiotics used commonly are penicillin, flucloxacillin, dicloxacillin, cefuroxime, or erythromycin. The usual intravenous antibiotics used are penicillin-based antibiotics (e.g., penicillin G or flucloxacillin) or cephalosporins (e.g., cefotaxime, ceftriaxone or cefazolin) for a few days. Sometimes oral probenecid is added to maintain antibiotic levels in the blood.

In situations where a broader antibiotic cover is required, for example a diabetic patient with a foot ulcer complicated by cellulitis, amoxicillin and clavulanic acid may be used. Clindamycin, sulfamethoxazole/trimethoprim, doxycycline, and vancomycin are alternative antibiotics in patients with serious penicillin or cephalosporin allergy, or where infection with methicillin-resistant *Staphylococcus aureus* is suspected.

Recurrent Cellulitis

Patients with recurrent cellulitis should:

- Avoid trauma, wear long sleeves and pants in high-risk activities e.g., gardening
- Keep skin clean and well moisturized, with nails well tended
- Avoid having blood tests taken from the affected limb
- Treat fungal infections of hands and feet early
- Keep swollen limbs elevated during rest periods to aid lymphatic circulation. Those with chronic lymphedema may benefit from compression garments.

Some patients with very frequent cellulitis may benefit from chronic suppressive antibiotic treatment with penicillin or erythromycin.

Impetigo

What Is Impetigo?

Impetigo is a bacterial skin infection. It is often called "school sores" because it most often affects children. It is quite contagious.

What Is The Cause Of Impetigo?

Streptococcus pyogenes and/or *Staphylococcus aureus* are the microorganisms responsible for impetigo.

Impetigo may be caught from someone else with impetigo or boils, or appear "out of the blue." It often starts at the site of a minor skin injury such as a graze, an insect bite, or scratched eczema.

What Does It Look Like?

Impetigo presents with pustules and round, oozing patches which grow larger day by day. There may be clear blisters (bullous impetigo) or golden yellow crusts. It most often occurs on exposed areas such as the hands and face, or in skin folds particularly the armpits.

Treatment

Treatment depends on the extent and severity of the infection.

- **Soak moist or crusted areas:** Soak a clean cloth in a mixture of half a cup of white vinegar in a liter of tepid water. Apply the compress to moist areas for about ten minutes several times a day. Gently wipe off the crusts.

- **Antiseptic or antibiotic ointment:** If an antiseptic (povidone iodine, hydrogen peroxide cream, chlorhexidine, and others) or antibiotic ointment (fusidic acid, mupirocin, or retapamulin) is prescribed, apply it two or three times a day to the affected areas and surrounding skin. Look carefully for new lesions to treat. Continue for several days after healing.

- **Oral antibiotics:** Oral antibiotics are recommended if the infection is extensive, proving slow to respond to topical antibiotics, or if the impetigo is recurrent. The preferred antibiotic is the penicillin antibiotic, flucloxacillin. The complete course should be taken, usually at least seven days.

- **Treat carrier sites:** If impetigo is proving hard to get rid of, the following measures may be useful:

- Apply an antibiotic ointment to the nostrils three times daily for seven days.

- Wash daily with antibacterial soap or cleanser.

- Soak in a bath containing a small amount of bleach.

- Take a prolonged course of oral antibiotics.

- Identify and treat the source of re-infection, i.e., another infected person or carrier. The nostrils of a household contact may be a carrier site for pathogenic bacteria, without that person having any sign of infection.

- **General measures:** During the infectious stage, i.e., while the impetigo is oozing or crusted:

  - Cover the affected areas.

  - Avoid close contact with others.

  - Affected children must stay away from school until crusts have dried out.

  - Use separate towels and washcloths.

  - Change and launder clothes and linen daily.

Necrotizing Fasciitis

What Is Necrotizing Fasciitis?

Necrotizing fasciitis is a very serious bacterial infection of the soft tissue and fascia (a sheath of tissue covering the muscle). The bacteria multiply and release toxins and enzymes that result in thrombosis (clotting) in the blood vessels. The result is destruction of the soft tissues and fascia.

There are three main types of necrotizing fasciitis:

- Type I (polymicrobial, i.e., more than one bacteria involved)

- Type II (due to hemolytic group A streptococcus)

- Type III (gas gangrene)

Bacteria causing type 1 necrotizing fasciitis include *Staphylococcus aureus*, *Haemophilus*, *Vibrio* and several other aerobic and anaerobic strains. It usually follows significant injury or surgery.

Type II necrotizing fasciitis has recently been sensationalized in the media and is commonly referred to as "flesh-eating" disease.

Type III is caused by *Clostridia perfringens* or less commonly *Clostridia septicum*. It usually follows significant injury or surgery and results in gas under the skin: this makes a crackling sound called crepitus.

How Do You Get Necrotizing Fasciitis?

Necrotizing fasciitis may occur in anyone, in fact, almost half of all known cases of streptococcal necrotizing fasciitis have occurred in young and previously healthy individuals. The disease may occur if the right set of conditions is present, these include:

- An opening in the skin that allows bacteria to enter the body. This may be very minor such as a small cut, graze, or pinprick or a large wound due to trauma or surgery. Sometimes no point of entry can be found.

- Direct contact with a person who is carrying the bacteria or the bacteria is already present elsewhere on the person.

- Particularly invasive strains of streptococci or other bacteria.

- In children, type II necrotizing fasciitis may complicate chickenpox.

- The risk is increased in those taking aspirin or non-steroidal anti-inflammatory drugs.

Those at increased risk of necrotizing fasciitis include diabetics, immunosuppressed individuals, obese people, drug abusers, and people with severe chronic illness.

What Are The Signs And Symptoms Of Necrotizing Fasciitis?

Signs and symptoms vary between individuals but often some or all of the following are present:

Symptoms appearing usually within 24 hours of a minor injury:

- Pain in the general area of the injury and worsening over time

- Flu-like symptoms such as nausea, fever, diarrhea, dizziness, and general malaise

- Intense thirst as body becomes dehydrated

Within three to four days of the initial symptoms the following may occur:

- Affected area starts to swell and may show a purplish rash

- Large dark marks form that turn into blisters filled with dark fluid

- Wound starts to die and area becomes blackened (necrosis)

- Severe pain

By about days 4–5, the patient is very ill with dangerously low blood pressure and high temperature. The infection has spread into the bloodstream and the body goes into toxic shock. The patient may have altered levels of consciousness or become totally unconscious.

What Treatment Is Available?

Once the diagnosis of necrotizing fasciitis is confirmed, treatment should be initiated without delay. Patients must be hospitalized, the causative organism(s) identified and treated with high dose intravenous antibiotics, often in an intensive care unit.

It is absolutely vital than an experienced surgeon urgently removes all dead tissue.

Treatment to raise blood pressure, hyperbaric oxygen, and intravenous immunoglobulin may also be necessary.

What Is The Likely Outcome?

If diagnosed and treated early, most patients will survive with minimal scarring. However if there is significant tissue loss, later skin grafting will be necessary and in some patients amputation of limbs is required to prevent death. Up to 25 percent of patients will die from the disease and complications such as renal failure and septicemia (blood poisoning) increase the likelihood of death.

Prompt diagnosis and treatment is essential to reducing the risk of death and disfigurement from necrotizing fasciitis.

Chapter 14

Pseudomonas Dermatitis (Hot Tub Rash)

This chapter addresses the most common questions regarding hot tub rash and healthy swimming.

Questions About Hot Tub Rash

What is hot tub rash?

Hot tub rash, or dermatitis, is an infection of the skin. Symptoms of hot tub rash include the following:

- Itchy spots on the skin that become a bumpy red rash.

- The rash is worse in areas that were previously covered by a swimsuit.

- Pus-filled blisters around hair follicles.

Hot tub rash can affect people of all ages.

What causes hot tub rash?

Hot tub rash is often caused by infection with the germ *Pseudomonas aeruginosa*.

This germ is common in the environment (for example, in the water and soil) and is microscopic, so it can't be seen with the naked eye.

About This Chapter: From "Hot Tub Rash (Pseudomonas Dermatitis/Folliculitis)," Centers for Disease Control And Prevention, May 26, 2011.

How is hot tub rash spread at recreational water venues?

Hot tub rash can occur if contaminated water comes in contact with skin for a long period of time.

The rash usually appears within a few days of being in a poorly maintained hot tub (or spa), but it can also appear within a few days after swimming in a poorly maintained pool or contaminated lake.

Most rashes clear up in a few days without medical treatment. However, if your rash lasts longer than a few days, consult your health care provider.

How do I protect myself and my family?

Because hot tubs have warmer water than pools, chlorine or other disinfectants used to kill germs (like *P. aeruginosa*) break down faster. This can increase the risk of hot tub rash infection for swimmers.

Here are some measures you can take to reduce the risk of hot tub rash:

- Remove your swimsuit and shower with soap after getting out of the water.

- Clean your swimsuit after getting out of the water.

- Ask your pool/hot tub operator if disinfectant (for example, chlorine) and pH levels are checked at least twice per day—hot tubs and pools with good disinfectant and pH control are less likely to spread germs.

- Use pool test strips to check the pool or hot tub yourself for adequate disinfectant (chlorine or bromine) levels. Centers for Disease Control and Prevention (CDC) recommends these standards for pools:

  - Pools: Free chlorine (1–3 parts per million or ppm)

  - Hot Tubs: Free chlorine (2–4 ppm) or bromine (4–6 ppm).

  - Both hot tubs and pools should have a pH level of 7.2–7.8.

  - If you find improper chlorine, bromine, and/or pH levels, tell the hot tub/pool operator or owner immediately.

Four Questions To Ask Your Hot Tub Operator

- What was the most recent health inspection score for the hot tub?

- Are disinfectant and pH levels checked at least twice per day?

- Are disinfectant and pH levels checked more often when the hot tub is being used by a lot of people?

- Are the following maintenance activities performed regularly:

  - Removal of the slime or biofilm layer by scrubbing and cleaning?

  - Replacement of the hot tub water filter according to manufacturer's recommendations?

  - Replacement of hot tub water?

Chapter 15

Lyme Disease

Lyme disease is caused by the bacterium *Borrelia burgdorferi* and is transmitted to humans through the bite of infected blacklegged ticks. Typical symptoms include fever, headache, fatigue, and a characteristic skin rash called erythema migrans. If left untreated, infection can spread to joints, the heart, and the nervous system. Lyme disease is diagnosed based on symptoms, physical findings (for example, rash), and the possibility of exposure to infected ticks; laboratory testing is helpful if used correctly and performed with validated methods. Most cases of Lyme disease can be treated successfully with a few weeks of antibiotics. Steps to prevent Lyme disease include using insect repellent, removing ticks promptly, applying pesticides, and reducing tick habitat. The ticks that transmit Lyme disease can occasionally transmit other tickborne diseases as well.

Preventing Tick Bites

Reducing exposure to ticks is the best defense against Lyme disease, Rocky Mountain spotted fever, and other tickborne infections. There are several steps you and your family can take to prevent and control Lyme disease:

While it is a good idea to take preventive measures against ticks year-round, be extra vigilant in warmer months (April–September) when ticks are most active.

Avoid Direct Contact With Ticks

- Avoid wooded and bushy areas with high grass and leaf litter.
- Walk in the center of trails.

About This Chapter: Excerpted from "Lyme Disease," October 1, 2012; "Preventing Tick Bites," and "Tick Removal," November 15, 2011; "Lyme Disease, Transmission," "Treatment," "Diagnosis and Testing," and "Signs and Symptoms of Lyme Disease," January 2013; Centers for Disease Control and Prevention (www.cdc.gov).

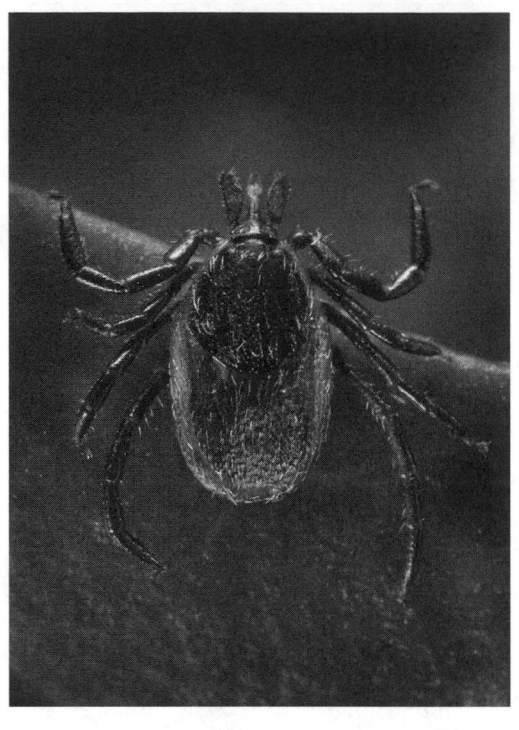

Figure 15.1. Western blacklegged tick. (Source: Centers for Disease Control and Prevention, Photo Credit: James Gathany, 2006).

Repel Ticks With DEET Or Permethrin

- Use repellents that contain 20 percent or more DEET (N, N-diethyl-m-toluamide) on the exposed skin for protection that lasts up to several hours. Always follow product instructions. Parents should apply this product to their children, avoiding hands, eyes, and mouth.

- Use products that contain permethrin on clothing. Treat clothing and gear, such as boots, pants, socks and tents. It remains protective through several washings. Pre-treated clothing is available and remains protective for up to 70 washings.

- Information about other repellents registered by the Environmental Protection Agency (EPA) may be found at http://cfpub.epa.gov/oppref/insect.

Find And Remove Ticks From Your Body

- Bathe or shower as soon as possible after coming indoors (preferably within two hours) to wash off and more easily find ticks that are crawling on you.

- Conduct a full-body tick check using a hand-held or full-length mirror to view all parts of your body upon return from tick-infested areas. Parents should check their children for ticks under the arms, in and around the ears, inside the belly button, behind the knees, between the legs, around the waist, and especially in their hair.

- Examine gear and pets. Ticks can ride into the home on clothing and pets, then attach to a person later, so carefully examine pets, coats, and day packs. Tumble clothes in a dryer on high heat for an hour to kill remaining ticks.

Tick Removal

If you find a tick attached to your skin, there's no need to panic. There are several tick removal devices on the market, but a plain set of fine-tipped tweezers will remove a tick quite effectively. Here's how to remove a tick:

- Use fine-tipped tweezers to grasp the tick as close to the skin's surface as possible.

- Pull upward with steady, even pressure. Don't twist or jerk the tick; this can cause the mouth-parts to break off and remain in the skin. If this happens, remove the mouth-parts with tweezers. If you are unable to remove the mouth easily with clean tweezers, leave it alone and let the skin heal.

- After removing the tick, thoroughly clean the bite area and your hands with rubbing alcohol, an iodine scrub, or soap and water.

Follow-Up

If you develop a rash or fever within several weeks of removing a tick, see your doctor. Be sure to tell the doctor about your recent tick bite, when the bite occurred, and where you most likely acquired the tick.

> Avoid folklore remedies such as "painting" the tick with nail polish or petroleum jelly, or using heat to make the tick detach from the skin. Your goal is to remove the tick as quickly as possible—not waiting for it to detach.

Lyme Disease Transmission

The Lyme disease bacterium, *B. burgdorferi*, is spread through the bite of infected ticks. The blacklegged tick (or deer tick, *Ixodes scapularis*) spreads the disease in the northeastern, mid-Atlantic, and north-central United States, and the western blacklegged tick (*Ixodes pacificus*) spreads the disease on the Pacific Coast.

Ticks can attach to any part of the human body but are often found in hard-to-see areas such as the groin, armpits, and scalp. In most cases, the tick must be attached for 36–48 hours or more before the Lyme disease bacterium can be transmitted.

Most humans are infected through the bites of immature ticks called nymphs. Nymphs are tiny (less than 2 mm) and difficult to see; they feed during the spring and summer months. Adult ticks can also transmit Lyme disease bacteria, but they are much larger and may be more likely to be discovered and removed before they have had time to transmit the bacteria. Adult *Ixodes* ticks are most active during the cooler months of the year.

Other Ways To Get Lyme Disease

- There is no evidence that Lyme disease is transmitted from person-to-person. For example, a person cannot get infected from touching, kissing or having sex with a person who has Lyme disease.

- Lyme disease acquired during pregnancy may lead to infection of the placenta and possible stillbirth; however, no negative effects on the fetus have been found when the mother receives appropriate antibiotic treatment. There are no reports of Lyme disease transmission from breast milk.

- Although no cases of Lyme disease have been linked to blood transfusion, scientists have found that the Lyme disease bacteria can live in blood that is stored for donation. Individuals being treated for Lyme disease with an antibiotic should not donate blood. Individuals who have completed antibiotic treatment for Lyme disease may be considered as potential blood donors. Information on the current criteria for blood donation is available on the Red Cross website at http://www.redcross.org/donate/give.

- Although dogs and cats can get Lyme disease, there is no evidence that they spread the disease directly to their owners. However, pets can bring infected ticks into your home or yard. Consider protecting your pet, and possibly yourself, through the use of tick control products for animals.

- You will not get Lyme disease from eating venison or squirrel meat, but in keeping with general food safety principles meat should always be cooked thoroughly. Note that hunting and dressing deer or squirrels may bring you into close contact with infected ticks.

- There is no credible evidence that Lyme disease can be transmitted through air, food, water, or from the bites of mosquitoes, flies, fleas, or lice.

- Ticks not known to transmit Lyme disease include Lone star ticks (*Amblyomma americanum*), the American dog tick (*Dermacentor variabilis*), the Rocky Mountain wood tick (*Dermacentor andersoni*), and the brown dog tick (*Rhipicephalus sanguineus*).

Signs And Symptoms Of Lyme Disease

If you had a tick bite, live in an area known for Lyme disease or have recently traveled to an area where it occurs, and observe any of these symptoms, you should seek medical attention!

Early Localized Stage (3–30 Days Post-Tick Bite)

- Red, expanding rash called erythema migrans (EM)

- Fatigue, chills, fever, headache, muscle and joint aches, and swollen lymph nodes

Some people may get these general symptoms in addition to an EM rash, but in others, these general symptoms may be the only evidence of infection.

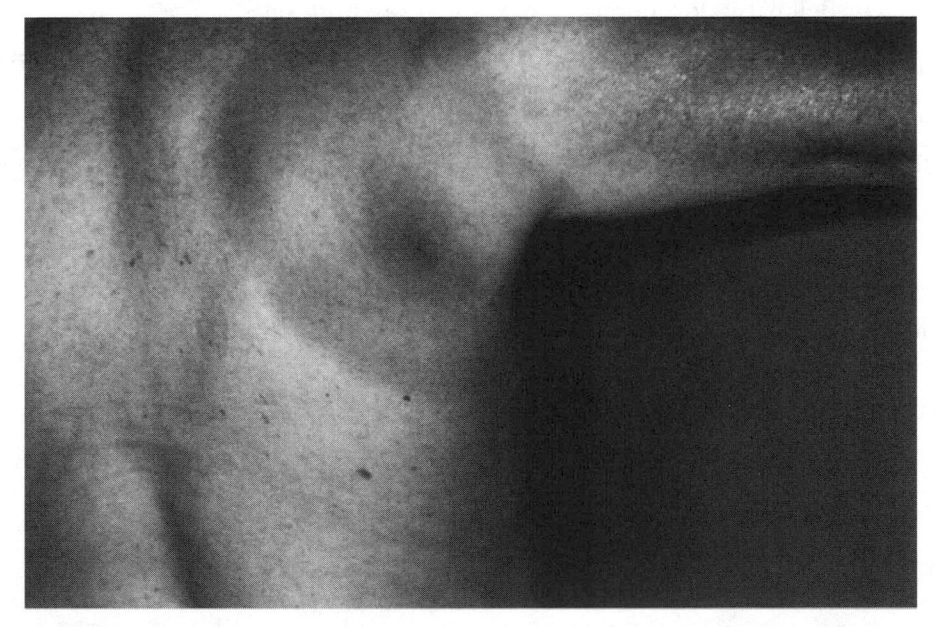

Figure 15.2. Bulls-eye rash. (Source: Centers for Disease Control and Prevention, Photo Credit: Anna Perez, 2005).

Some people get a small bump or redness at the site of a tick bite that goes away in 1–2 days, like a mosquito bite. This is not a sign that you have Lyme disease. However, ticks can spread other organisms that may cause a different type of rash. For example, southern tick-associated rash illness (STARI) causes a rash with a very similar appearance.

Erythema migrans or **bull's-eye rash** can include the following features:

- Rash occurs in approximately 70–80 percent of infected persons1 and begins at the site of a tick bite after a delay of 3–30 days (average is about seven days).

- Rash gradually expands over a period of several days, and can reach up to 12 inches (30 cm) across. Parts of the rash may clear as it enlarges, resulting in a bull's-eye appearance.

- Rash usually feels warm to the touch but is rarely itchy or painful.

- EM lesions may appear on any area of the body.

Early Disseminated Stage (Days To Weeks Post-Tick Bite)

Untreated, the infection may spread from the site of the bite to other parts of the body, producing an array of specific symptoms that may come and go, including the following:

- Additional EM lesions in other areas of the body

- Facial or Bell palsy (loss of muscle tone on one or both sides of the face)

- Severe headaches and neck stiffness due to meningitis (inflammation of the spinal cord)

- Pain and swelling in the large joints (such as knees)

- Shooting pains that may interfere with sleep

- Heart palpitations and dizziness due to changes in heartbeat

Many of these symptoms will resolve over a period of weeks to months, even without treatment. However, lack of treatment can result in additional complications.

Lyme Disease Diagnosis And Treatment

Lyme disease is diagnosed based on two factors:

- Signs and symptoms

- A history of possible exposure to infected blacklegged ticks

Laboratory blood tests are helpful if used correctly and performed with validated methods. Laboratory tests are not recommended for patients who do not have symptoms typical of

Lyme disease. Just as it is important to correctly diagnose Lyme disease when a patient has it, it is important to avoid misdiagnosis and treatment of Lyme disease when the true cause of the illness is something else.

Laboratory Testing

Laboratory testing can be an important aid in the diagnosis of Lyme disease. Proper use and interpretation of laboratory tests requires an understanding of the type of test, the stage of illness, and the underlying likelihood that the patient has the disease.

Like blood tests for many other infectious diseases, the test for Lyme disease measures antibodies made by white blood cells in response to infection. It can take several weeks after infection for the body to produce sufficient antibodies to be detected. Therefore, patients tested during the first few weeks of illness will often test negative. In contrast, patients who have had Lyme disease for longer than 4–6 weeks, especially those with later stages of illness involving the brain or the joints, will almost always test positive. A patient who has been ill for months or years and has a negative test almost certainly does not have Lyme disease as the cause of their symptoms.

Because all laboratory tests can sometimes give falsely positive results, it is important when faced with a positive result to consider the underlying likelihood that a patient has the disease. If a patient has not been in an area where Lyme disease is common or their symptoms are atypical, positive results are more likely to be false positives. Similarly, if a patient is tested numerous times and only rarely tests positive, it is likely that the positive result is a false positive.

Treatment

Patients treated with appropriate antibiotics in the early stages of Lyme disease usually recover rapidly and completely. Antibiotics commonly used for oral treatment include doxycycline, amoxicillin, or cefuroxime axetil. Patients with certain neurological or cardiac forms of illness may require intravenous treatment with drugs such as ceftriaxone or penicillin. For detailed recommendations on treatment, consult the 2006 Guidelines for treatment developed by the Infectious Diseases Society of America.

Approximately 10-20 percent of patients (particularly those who were diagnosed later), following appropriate antibiotic treatment, may have persistent or recurrent symptoms and are considered to have post-treatment Lyme disease syndrome (PTLDS). The National Institutes of Health (NIH) has funded several studies on the treatment of Lyme disease which show that most patients recover when treated with a few weeks of antibiotics taken by mouth. For details on research into what is sometimes referred to as "chronic Lyme disease" and long-term treatment trials sponsored by NIH, visit the NIH Lyme Disease website at http://health.nih .gov/topic/LymeDisease.

Chapter 16

Cold Sores And Canker Sores

Cold Sores (HSV-1)

Neal knew something weird was going on. A few days before, his lip started tingling and felt a little numb. He didn't pay much attention to it then, but now there was a certain throbbing something on his lip and it wasn't pretty. At first Neal thought it was a zit because it was red and tender, but then it blistered and opened up. Neal had a cold sore.

Maybe you've heard of a fever blister—a cold sore is the same thing. They're pretty common and lots of people get them. So what exactly are cold sores and what causes them?

What's A Cold Sore?

Cold sores, which are small and somewhat painful blisters that usually show up on or around a person's lips, are caused by **herpes simplex virus-1 (HSV-1)**. But they don't just show up on the lips. They can sometimes be inside the mouth, on the face, or even inside or on the nose. These places are the most common, but sores can appear anywhere on the body, including the genital area.

Genital herpes isn't typically caused by HSV-1; it's caused by another type of the herpes simplex virus called **herpes simplex virus-2 (HSV-2)** and is spread by sexual contact. But even though HSV-1 typically causes sores around the mouth and HSV-2 causes genital sores, these viruses can cause sores in either place.

About This Chapter: "Cold Sores (HSV-1)," October 2010, and "Canker Sores," January 2013, reprinted with permission from www.kidshealth.org. This information was provided by KidsHealth®, one of the largest resources online for medically reviewed health information written for parents, kids, and teens. For more articles like this, visit www.KidsHealth.org, or www.TeensHealth.org. Copyright © 1995-2013 The Nemours Foundation. All rights reserved.

What Causes A Cold Sore?

HSV-1 is very common — if you have it, chances are you picked it up when you were a kid. Most people who are infected with the herpes simplex virus got it during their preschool years, most likely from close contact with someone who has it or getting kissed by an adult with the virus.

Although a person who has HSV-1 doesn't always have sores, the virus stays in the body and there's no permanent cure.

When someone gets infected with HSV-1, the virus makes its way through the skin and into a group of nerve cells called a **ganglion** (pronounced: **gang**-glee-in). The virus moves in here, takes a long snooze, and every now and then decides to wake up and cause a cold sore. But not everyone who gets the herpes simplex virus develops cold sores. In some people, the virus stays dormant (asleep) permanently.

What causes the virus to "wake up" or reactivate? The truth is, no one knows for sure. A person doesn't necessarily have to have a cold to get a cold sore—they can be brought on by other infections, fever, stress, sunlight, cold weather, hormone changes in menstruation or pregnancy, tooth extractions, and certain foods and drugs. In a lot of people, the cause is unpredictable.

Here's how a cold sore develops:

- The herpes simplex virus-1, which has been lying dormant in the body, reactivates or "wakes up."
- The virus travels toward the area where the cold sore decides to show up (like a person's lip) via the nerve endings.
- The area below the skin's surface, where the cold sore is going to appear, starts to tingle, itch, or burn.
- A red bump appears in the area about a day or so after the tingling.
- The bump blisters and turns into a cold sore.
- After a few days, the cold sore dries up and a yellow crust appears in its place.
- The scab-like yellow crust falls off and leaves behind a pinkish area where it once was.
- The redness fades away as the body heals and sends the herpes simplex virus back to "sleep."

How Do Cold Sores Spread?

Cold sores are really contagious. If you have a cold sore, it's very easy to infect another person with HSV-1. The virus spreads through direct contact—through skin contact or contact with oral or genital secretions (like through kissing). Although the virus is most contagious when a sore is present, it can still be passed on even if you can't see a sore. HSV-1 can also be spread by sharing a cup, eating utensils, or lip balm or lipstick with someone who has it.

In addition, if you or your partner gets cold sores on the mouth, the herpes simplex virus-1 can be transmitted during oral sex and cause herpes in the genital area.

Herpes simplex virus-1 also can spread if a person touches the cold sore and then touches a mucous membrane or an area of the skin with a cut on it. Mucous membranes are the moist, protective linings made of tissue that are found in certain areas of your body like your nose, eyes, mouth, and vagina. So it's best to not mess with a cold sore—don't pick, pinch, or squeeze it.

Actually, it's a good idea to not even touch active cold sores. If you do touch an active cold sore, don't touch other parts of your body. Be especially careful about touching your eyes—if it gets into the eyes, HSV-1 can cause a lot of damage. Wash your hands as soon as possible. In fact, if you have a cold sore or you're around someone with a cold sore, try to wash your hands frequently.

If they aren't taken care of properly, cold sores can develop into bacterial skin infections. And they can actually be dangerous for people whose immune systems are weakened (such as infants and people who have cancer or HIV/AIDS) as well as those with eczema. For people with any of these conditions, an infection triggered by a cold sore can actually be life threatening.

How Are Cold Sores Diagnosed And Treated?

Cold sores normally go away on their own within 7 to 10 days. And although no medications can make the infection go away, prescription drugs and creams are available that can shorten the length of the outbreak and make the cold sore less painful.

If you have a cold sore, it's important to see your doctor if:

- You have another health condition that has weakened your immune system
- The sores don't heal by themselves within 7 to 10 days
- You get cold sores frequently
- You have signs of a bacterial infection, such as fever, pus, or spreading redness

To make yourself more comfortable when you have cold sores, you can apply ice or anything cool to the area. You also can take an over-the-counter pain reliever, such as acetaminophen or ibuprofen.

Canker Sores

What's A Canker Sore?

If you've ever had those open, shallow sores in your mouth and taken a gulp of orange juice, you know what a pain canker sores can be. Canker sores are fairly common: About one in five people get them on a regular basis. The good news is, they usually go away on their own without treatment.

Canker sores (also known as **aphthous ulcers**) only happen inside the mouth. You can get them on or under the tongue and on the inside of the cheeks and lips—the parts of the mouth that can move. They usually pop up alone, but sometimes they show up in small clusters.

Signs It's A Canker Sore

Your mouth might tingle or burn before a canker sore appears. Soon, a small red bump rises. Then after a day or so it bursts, leaving an open, shallow white or yellowish wound with a red border. The sores are often painful and can be up to half an inch across, although most of them are much smaller. A person who has canker sores doesn't usually have the fever or swollen lymph nodes that can show up with some other kinds of sores. Aside from the annoying pain in the mouth, you'll generally feel OK.

The good news is that canker sores are *not* contagious like some other mouth sores, such as cold sores. You can't get canker sores by sharing food or kissing someone.

If you have a sore and you're wondering if it's a cold sore or a canker sore, just look at where it shows up: Cold sores usually appear *outside* the mouth, around the lips, chin, or nostrils. Canker sores are always found *inside* the mouth.

You can also get spots in your mouth when you have an infection like chickenpox or measles. In some cases of these diseases, the rash actually spreads into the mouth. If you have chickenpox or measles, you'll find spots on other parts of your body as well, so you'll know they're not canker sores.

Causes

Canker sores usually begin showing up between the ages of 10 and 20, although they can happen at any time in a person's life. No one knows exactly what causes them. One thing that doctors have noticed is that although the sores are not contagious, they can run in families. That means if your parents or siblings get canker sores, the genes you share with them make it more likely that you'll develop the sores, too.

There may be a connection between canker sores and stress. If you get canker sores around exam time or some other big event in your life, it may be a sign of how much stress you're under. In addition, about twice as many women as men get them. Doctors think that may be due to the differences in male and female hormones, especially because women often get them during certain times in their menstrual cycle.

Some research suggests that using products containing sodium lauryl sulfate (SLS) can be associated with canker sores. SLS is a foaming agent found in most toothpastes and mouthwashes. Finally, not getting the right nutrition, such as not getting enough iron or vitamin B12, may also contribute to some cases of canker sores.

What You Can Do

Most canker sores will heal on their own in a few days to a couple of weeks. While you're waiting for them to disappear, you can take over-the-counter pain relievers like ibuprofen or acetaminophen for the pain. You'll also want to watch what you eat. Spicy foods and acidic foods such as lemons or tomatoes can be extremely painful on these open wounds. Stay away from hard, scratchy, or crunchy foods like nuts, toast, pretzels, or potato chips for a while. They can poke or rub the sore.

Be careful when you brush your teeth. Brush and rinse with toothpastes and mouthwashes that don't contain sodium lauryl sulfate. And avoid brushing the sore itself with a toothbrush, which will make it worse.

There are lots of "home remedies" for canker sores out there, but no evidence to show that they help sores heal faster. If you have canker sores that do not get better after a few weeks, if the sores keep coming back, or if they make you feel so sick that you don't want to eat, call your doctor or dentist. He or she may prescribe a topical medicine or special mouthwash to help heal the sores.

For medications that are applied directly to the sore, first blot the area dry with a tissue. Use a cotton swab to apply a small amount of the medication, and do not eat or drink for at least 30 minutes to make sure that the medicine is not immediately washed away.

In some cases, doctors may want to do blood tests to find out if another condition—such as a vitamin deficiency, a problem with your immune system, or even a food allergy—could be contributing to the sores.

Although they can certainly be a pain, in most cases canker sores aren't serious and should go away on their own.

Chapter 17

Papillomaviruses And Skin Warts

What Are Warts?

Warts are tiny skin infections caused by viruses of the human papillomavirus (HPV) family. Although kids get warts most often, teens and adults can get them, too. Sometimes warts are sexually transmitted and appear in the genital area, but most warts affect the fingers, hands, and feet.

Some people appear to be more susceptible to warts than others. In fact, some people never get them. Doctors aren't really sure why this is and think it may be that some people's immune systems make them less likely to get the viruses that cause warts.

These viruses are passed from person to person by close physical contact. Having a tiny scratch or cut can make someone more vulnerable to getting warts.

What Are The Signs And Symptoms?

If you find a small, hard bump on your skin that has a rough surface similar to that of cauliflower, it's probably a wart. Warts can look pink, white, or brown, and can contain tiny spots inside that look like black specks. Warts can affect any part of the skin, but are most often found on the extremities—fingers, hands, and feet.

Warts are usually painless, except for those on the soles of the feet. These are called plantar warts, and if you have one it can feel like walking on a small pebble. Warts on the palms of the hands or soles of the feet may appear level rather than raised.

About This Chapter "Warts," November 2010, reprinted with permission from www.kidshealth.org. This information was provided by KidsHealth®, one of the largest resources online for medically reviewed health information written for parents, kids, and teens. For more articles like this, visit www.KidsHealth.org, or www.TeensHealth.org. Copyright © 1995-2012 The Nemours Foundation. All rights reserved.

Sometimes warts can itch or bleed. They may also become infected with bacteria (from scratching or picking) and become red, hot, or tender.

Can I Prevent Warts?

There is no way to prevent warts, but it's always a good idea to wash your skin regularly and well. If you cut or scratch your skin, be sure to use soap and water because open wounds are more susceptible to warts and other infections.

It's also a good idea to wear waterproof sandals or flip-flops in public showers, locker rooms, and around public pools (this also can help protect against other infections, like athlete's foot).

If you do have a wart, don't rub, scratch, or pick at it or you may spread the virus to another part of your body or cause the wart to become infected.

How Long Before Symptoms Appear?

The length of time between when someone is exposed to an HPV virus and a wart appears varies, but warts can grow very slowly and may take many months to develop.

How Long Do Warts Last?

Warts are different in different people. In time, many warts disappear on their own.

With treatment, warts can usually be removed within a few weeks, but they may come back if the virus causing them stays in the skin.

When Should I Call A Doctor?

Although many warts disappear on their own with time, it's a good idea to show your wart to a doctor, who can recommend a treatment method if you need one.

If you discover a wart on your face or on your genital area, call your doctor. He or she can determine the best treatment for those areas, which are very sensitive.

How Are Warts Treated?

Warts can be treated in various ways:

- **Over-the-counter medications** contain acids that are applied to the wart. The acids are peeling agents that remove the dead skin cells of the wart and cause the wart to eventually fall off. OTC treatments shouldn't be used on the face or genitals without consulting a doctor first as some of them may damage the skin.

- **Cryosurgery** (pronounced: kry-o-**sur**-juh-ree) is where a doctor freezes the wart with liquid nitrogen. This treatment is usually done in the doctor's office.

- **Laser surgery** may be used for warts that are hard to remove.

Within a few days after treatment by a doctor, a small wart will usually fall off, although you may need more than one treatment. Treatment may take longer for larger warts. Over-the-counter treatments may take longer than the doctor's office treatments, but can be used as initial treatment on the hands or feet. Your doctor may also tell you to use OTC treatments after you've had an in-office procedure.

What Can I Do To Help Myself Feel Better?

If you have a simple wart on a finger or toe, you can try to remove it with an over-the-counter medication. These include liquids or pads containing medication that work by chemically removing the skin affected by the wart virus.

Because these are strong chemicals, you should follow the directions and use them with care to prevent removing healthy skin. Keep the chemicals away from your eyes, and wash your hands thoroughly after treating the area.

Chapter 18

Human Papillomavirus (HPV) And Genital Warts

Human Papillomavirus

Human papillomavirus (HPV) is one of the most common causes of sexually transmitted disease (STD) in the world. Health experts estimate there are more cases of genital HPV infection than any other STD in the United States. According to the Centers for Disease Control and Prevention, approximately 6 million new cases of sexually transmitted HPV infections are reported every year. At least 20 million people in this country are already infected.

Genital Warts

Genital warts (sometimes called *condylomata acuminata* or venereal warts) are the most easily recognized sign of genital HPV infection. Many people, however, have a genital HPV infection without genital warts.

Genital warts are soft, moist, or flesh colored and appear in the genital area within weeks or months after infection. They sometimes appear in clusters that resemble cauliflower-like bumps, and are either raised or flat, small or large. Genital warts can show up in women on the vulva and cervix, and inside and surrounding the vagina and anus. In men, genital warts can appear on the scrotum or penis. There are cases where genital warts have been found on the thigh and groin.

About This Chapter: Excerpted from "Human Papilloma Virus (HPV) And Genital Warts," National Institute of Allergy and Infectious Diseases (www.niaid.nih.gov), May 12, 2010.

Cause

More than 100 different types of HPV exist, most of which are harmless. About 30 types are spread through sexual contact and are classified as either low risk or high risk.

Some types of HPV cause genital warts—single or multiple bumps that appear in the genital areas of men and women including the vagina, cervix, vulva (area outside of the vagina), penis, and rectum. These are considered low-risk types.

High-risk types of HPV may cause abnormal Pap smear results. They could lead to cancers of the cervix, vulva, vagina, anus, or penis.

Prevention

The best way to prevent getting an HPV infection is to avoid direct contact with the virus, which is transmitted by skin-to-skin contact. If you or your sexual partner has warts that are visible in the genital area, you should avoid any skin-to skin and sexual contact until the warts are treated.

Two HPV vaccines, Gardasil and Cervarix, are approved by the Food and Drug Administration. Both vaccines are highly effective in preventing persistent infection with HPV types 16 and 18, two "high-risk" HPVs that cause most (70 percent) of cervical cancers. Gardasil is also effective against types 6 and 11, which cause virtually all (90 percent) of genital warts.

Both vaccines are licensed, safe, and effective for females ages 9 through 26 years. The Centers for Disease Control and Prevention (CDC) recommends that all girls who are 11 or 12 years old get the three doses of either brand of HPV vaccine to protect against cervical cancer and precancer.

Gardasil is also licensed for boys and young men ages 9 through 26 years. Males may choose to get this vaccine to prevent genital warts.

Neither Gardasil nor Cervarix has been proven to provide complete protection against persistent infection with other HPV types, some of which also can cause cervical cancer. Therefore, about 30 percent of cervical cancers and 10 percent of genital warts will not be prevented by the current vaccines. HPV vaccines do not prevent other sexually transmitted diseases, nor do they treat HPV infection or cervical cancer.

For federal HPV vaccine recommendations, go to the CDC Advisory Committee on Immunization Practices website at www.cdc.gov/vaccines/recs/acip. In addition, the National

Cancer Institute and CDC have more information on the HPV vaccine at www.cancer.gov/cancertopics/hpv-vaccines and www.cdc.gov/vaccines/vpd-vac/hpv/default.htm, respectively.

Historically, research studies have not confirmed that male latex condoms prevent transmission of HPV. Recent studies, however, demonstrate that consistent condom use by male partners suggests strong protection against low-risk and high-risk types of HPV infection in women. Unfortunately, many people who don't have symptoms don't know that they can spread the virus to an uninfected partner.

Chapter 19

Varicella (Chickenpox And Shingles)

Chickenpox (varicella) is a common, preventable childhood infection caused by the varicella-zoster virus. It's most common in children and is usually mild, but can be very uncomfortable. When adults get it they can be very sick.

Chickenpox is very dangerous for people with immune system problems like leukemia or for people who are taking drugs that weaken the immune system (such as steroids).

What are the symptoms?

- Chickenpox begins with a fever.

- Within one to two days people get a rash that can be very itchy.

- It starts with red spots that soon turn into fluid-filled blisters.

- Some people have only a few blisters. Others can have as many as 500.

- These blisters dry and form scabs in four or five days.

How is it spread?

Chickenpox spreads easily. It can spread from two days before the rash appears but is most contagious 12 to 24 hours before the rash appears, so it's easy to spread it without knowing. It usually develops two to three weeks after contact with an infected person.

About This Chapter: The information in this chapter is reprinted with permission from: Canadian Paediatric Society, Infectious Diseases and Immunization Committee. Chickenpox. For more information, please visit www.caringforkids.cps.ca. © Canadian Paediatric Society, updated September 2011.

- It spreads from person to person through direct contact with the virus. You can get chickenpox if you touch a blister or the liquid from a blister. You can also get chickenpox if you touch the spit of a person who has it.

- The virus enters the body by the nose or mouth.

- It can also spread through the air.

- A pregnant woman with chickenpox can pass it on to her baby before birth.

- Mothers with chickenpox can also give it to their newborn babies after birth.

The only way to stop the spread of the virus from person to person is to stop infected people from sharing the same room or house, which isn't practical.

Chickenpox doesn't spread through indirect contact. That means it doesn't live on objects like sheets, counters, or toys.

Is there a vaccine against chickenpox?

Yes.

- Children should get two shots for chickenpox: the first when they are 12 to 18 months old and a second "booster" shot when they are four to six years old.

- Teens (13 years and older) who have never had chickenpox should get two shots, at least four weeks apart.

What is shingles?

Shingles happens in people who have already had chickenpox, usually many years later. It looks like chickenpox and is caused by the same virus. But it usually appears on only one part of the body. Shingles is contagious, but is less contagious than chickenpox because it doesn't spread through the air.

- You can catch chickenpox from someone with shingles through contact with their saliva or their skin rash.

- You cannot get shingles from someone with chickenpox.

Can you have chickenpox twice?

In most cases, you can only get chickenpox once. This is called lifelong immunity. But in rare cases, a person might get it again, especially if he or she was very young the first time.

How is chickenpox prevented?

The best way protection from chickenpox is vaccination.

If a child is not yet vaccinated and comes in contact with another child or family member who has chickenpox, he may still be protected if he is vaccinated right away.

If a child has chickenpox, it will probably spread to other members of the household who have not already had chickenpox or the vaccine.

How can chickenpox be treated?

- If you get chickenpox, do not take or give aspirin [acetylsalicylic acid (ASA)] or any products that contain aspirin. Taking aspirin increases the risk of getting Reye's syndrome. This severe illness can damage the liver and brain. If you want to control your fever, use acetaminophen (Tylenol, Tempra, Panadol, and others).

- Don't scratch. Scratching can cause infection from bacteria that get into the skin. Adding baking soda to the bathwater can be soothing. Your doctor may recommend a cream to help reduce the itch.

When should I call the doctor?

- A fever lasts more than two days and is over 38.5°C (101.3°F).

- A new fever develops after the first couple of days. That is, the fever goes away for a day or so and returns.

- You develop a skin infection and look ill, especially along with high fever. Your doctor will decide if bacterial infection has developed that needs antibiotics.

- A chickenpox spot becomes enlarged, red, or very sore.

- You seem very ill.

- You have an immune system disorder. The doctor can give a special type of immune globulin (VZIG) with a large number of antibodies to help prevent infection, or early treatment with an antiviral drug.

Can someone with chickenpox go to child care or school?

Many schools and daycare centers have policies that require children with chickenpox to stay home for five days after their rash appears. The goal is to protect other children from the disease. Unfortunately, this does not stop chickenpox from spreading.

Chickenpox is contagious from two days before the rash appears, and most infectious from 12 to 24 hours before the rash appears. It spreads through the air, not just by direct contact with the rash. Exclusion policies (policies that require someone with chickenpox to stay home for a period of time) don't work because by the time it's known that someone has chickenpox, it has already been passed on to others.

If someone with chickenpox is too sick to take part in regular activities, or if he has a fever, he should stay home. Many children with mild chickenpox are otherwise well. For mild cases (low fever for a short period of time and only a little rash, less than 30 spots) children can go to child care or school as long as they feel well enough to take part in regular activities, even if they still have the rash.

What about pregnant women?

Pregnant women can develop severe chickenpox. Most adult women are already protected against chickenpox by antibodies in their blood. Women who have not had chickenpox should ask their doctors about whether vaccination would be appropriate.

If you are pregnant and have not had chickenpox, or if you have not lived in the same house with someone who has had chickenpox or shingles, call your doctor right away if you are exposed to chickenpox. Your doctor may want to give you a special type of immune globulin (VZIG) injection to help prevent you from getting a severe infection.

Women who catch chickenpox early in pregnancy have a very small chance of it harming their unborn infants.

Chapter 20

Parvovirus B19 (Fifth Disease)

Fifth Disease Overview

Fifth disease is a mild rash illness caused by parvovirus B19. This disease is also called *erythema infectiosum*. It is more common in children than adults. A person usually gets sick within 4 to 14 days (sometimes up to 20 days) after getting infected with parvovirus B19. About 20 percent of children and adults who get infected with this virus will not have any symptoms.

Signs And Symptoms

The first symptoms of fifth disease are usually mild and nonspecific. The first symptoms of fifth disease are usually the following:

- Fever
- Runny nose
- Headache

Then, you can get a rash on your face and body. After several days, you may get a red rash on your face. This is called slapped cheek rash. This rash is the most recognized feature of fifth disease. It is more common in children than adults. Some people may get a second rash a few days later on their chest, back, buttocks, or arms and legs. The rash may be itchy, especially on the soles of the feet. The rash can vary in intensity and may come and go for several weeks. It usually goes away in 7 to 10 days, but it can last several weeks. As the rash starts to go away, it may look lacy.

About This Chapter: From "Parvovirus B19 And Fifth Disease," Centers for Disease Control and Prevention (www.cdc.gov), February 14, 2012.

You may also have painful or swollen joints. People with fifth disease can also develop pain and swelling in their joints (polyarthropathy syndrome). This is more common in adults, especially women. Some adults with fifth disease may only have painful joints, usually in the hands, feet, or knees, but no other symptoms. The joint pain usually lasts one to three weeks, but it can last for months or longer. It usually goes away without any long-term problems.

Transmission

Parvovirus B19 spreads through respiratory secretions (such as saliva, sputum, or nasal mucus) when an infected person coughs or sneezes. You are most contagious when it seems like you have just a cold and before you get the rash or joint pain and swelling. After you get the rash, you are probably not contagious. So, it is usually safe for you to go back to school.

The contagious period for fifth disease is different from many other rash illnesses. For example, people with measles can spread the measles virus when they have the rash. However, people with fifth disease who weakened immune systems may be contagious for a longer amount of time.

Parvovirus B19 can also spread through blood or blood products. A pregnant woman who is infected with parvovirus B19 can pass the virus to her baby.

Diagnosis

Healthcare providers can often diagnose fifth disease just by seeing slapped cheek rash on a patient's face. A blood test can also be done to determine if you arc susceptible or immune to parvovirus B19 infection or if you were recently infected.

Once you recover from fifth disease, you develop immunity that generally protects you from parvovirus B19 infection in the future.

People with fifth disease are most contagious before they get rash or joint pain and swelling.

Prevention And Treatment

Prevention

People with fifth disease are most contagious when it seems like they have just a cold and before they get the rash or joint pain and swelling.

You can reduce your chance of being infected with parvovirus B19 or infecting others by taking these precautions:

- Washing your hands often with soap and water
- Covering your mouth and nose when you cough or sneeze
- Not touching your eyes, nose, or mouth
- Avoiding close contact with people who are sick
- Staying home when you are sick

After you get the rash, you are probably not contagious. So, it is usually safe for you to return to school.

All healthcare providers and patients should follow strict infection control practices to prevent parvovirus B19 from spreading.

For information about hand washing, see "CDC's Clean Hands Save Lives!" at http://www.cdc.gov/handwashing/.

Treatment

Fifth disease is usually mild and will go away on its own. Children and adults who are otherwise healthy usually recover completely.

Treatment usually involves relieving symptoms, such as fever, itching, and joint pain and swelling.

People who have complications from fifth disease should see their healthcare provider for medical treatment.

There is no vaccine or medicine that can prevent parvovirus B19 infection.

Complications

Fifth disease is usually mild for children and adults who are otherwise healthy. But, for some people, fifth disease cause serious health complications.

People with weakened immune systems caused by leukemia, cancer, organ transplants, or HIV infection are at risk for serious complications from fifth disease. It can cause chronic anemia that requires medical treatment.

Chapter 21

Tinea Infections: Ringworm, Jock Itch, And Athlete's Foot

Ringworm

Although their names—ringworm, jock itch, and athlete's foot—may sound funny, if you're a teen with one of these skin infections, you're probably not laughing. If you've ever had one, you know that all of these can produce some pretty unpleasant symptoms.

The good news is that tinea, the name for this category of common skin infections, is generally easy to treat.

What is ringworm?

Ringworm, which isn't a worm at all, can affect not only the skin, but also the nails and scalp.

Ringworm of the skin starts as a red, scaly patch or bump. Ringworm tends to be very itchy and uncomfortable. Over time, it may begin to look like a ring or a series of rings with raised, bumpy, scaly borders (the center is often clear). This ring pattern gave ringworm its name, but not every person who's infected develops the rings.

When ringworm affects the feet it's known as athlete's foot, and the rash, which is usually between a person's toes, appears patchy. In fact, the rashes a person gets with athlete's foot and jock itch may not look like rings at all—they may be red, scaly patches.

About This Chapter: "Tinea (Ringworm, Jock Itch, Athlete's Foot)," October 2011, reprinted with permission from www.kidshealth.org. This information was provided by KidsHealth®, one of the largest resources online for medically reviewed health information written for parents, kids, and teens. For more articles like this, visit www.KidsHealth.org or www.TeensHealth.org. Copyright © 1995-2012 The Nemours Foundation. All rights reserved.

Ringworm of the scalp may start as a small sore that resembles a pimple before becoming patchy, flaky, or scaly. It may cause some hair to fall out or break into stubbles. It can also cause the place where the infection is to become swollen, tender, and red.

Ringworm of the nails may affect one or more nails on a person's hands or feet. The nails may become thick, white or yellowish, and brittle. Ringworm of the nails is not too common before puberty, though.

Can I prevent ringworm?

The most common sources of the fungi that cause tinea infections are other people. Ringworm is contagious and is easily spread from one person to another, so avoid touching an infected area on another person. It's also possible to become infected from contact with animals, like cats and dogs.

It can be difficult to avoid ringworm because the dermatophyte fungi are very common. To protect yourself against infection, it can help to wear flip-flops on your feet in the locker room shower or at the pool, and to wash sports clothing regularly. Because fungi are on your skin, it's important to shower after contact sports and to wash your hands often, especially after touching pets.

If you discover a red, patchy, itchy area that you think may be ringworm, call your doctor.

How is ringworm treated?

Fortunately, ringworm is fairly easy to diagnose and treat. Doctors usually can diagnose ringworm based on how it looks, but sometimes will scrape off a small sample of the flaky infected skin to test for fungus.

If you do have ringworm, your doctor will recommend an antifungal medication. A topical ointment or cream usually takes care of skin infections, but ringworm of the scalp or nails requires oral antifungal medication. Your doctor will decide which treatment is best for you.

Jock Itch

Game over! It was a hard-fought match, and Pete's team just won in the final seconds. Now, as he basks in the afterglow of sweet victory, he thinks about all the great things he's going to get for his sweaty effort—admiring glances, bragging rights, a medal, a trophy, maybe even a mention in the local paper.

But he's feeling a little itchy and uncomfortable in an area due south. And it's starting to burn. Yes, it's something else Pete got for his athletic efforts—jock itch.

What is jock itch?

Jock itch is a pretty common fungal infection of the groin and upper thighs. It's part of a group of fungal skin infections called tinea. The medical name for jock itch is **tinea cruris** (pronounced: **tih**-nee-uh krur-us).

Jock itch, like other tinea infections, is caused by several types of mold-like fungi called dermatophytes (pronounced: dur-**mah**-tuh-fites). All of us have microscopic fungi and bacteria living on our bodies, and dermatophytes are among them. Dermatophytes live on the dead tissues of your skin, hair, and nails and thrive in warm, moist areas like the insides of the thighs. So, when the groin area gets sweaty and isn't dried properly, it provides a perfect environment for the fungi to multiply and thrive.

Who gets jock itch?

You don't have to be a jock to get that itch down south. Jock itch is so named because mostly athletes get it. But it can affect anyone who tends to sweat a lot. It most often affects guys, but girls can get it, too.

Some things can make jock itch more likely to develop. These include lots of sweating while playing sports, hot and humid weather, friction from wearing tight clothes for extended periods (like bathing suits), and sharing clothes with others.

People who have certain health conditions, such as obesity, diabetes mellitus, or other diseases that cause problems with the immune system, are also more likely to develop it.

What are the signs and symptoms?

Jock itch is usually less severe than other tinea infections. If it's not treated, though, it can last for weeks or months. Symptoms of jock itch include the following:

- A circular, red, raised rash with elevated edges
- Itching, chafing, or burning in the groin, thigh, or anal area
- Skin redness in the groin, thigh, or anal area
- Flaking, peeling, or cracking skin

How do I get rid of it?

Jock itch usually responds to self-care: Over-the-counter antifungal creams, powders, and sprays will probably clear it up. Sometimes, though, a person may need to see a doctor for a prescription antifungal cream.

The Basics On Tinea Infections

Tinea (pronounced: **tih**-nee-uh) is the medical name for a group of related skin infections, including athlete's foot, jock itch, and ringworm. They're caused by several types of mold-like fungi called **dermatophytes** (pronounced: der-**mah**-tuh-fites) that live on the dead tissues of the skin, hair, and nails.

When it comes to healing a fungal infection, it's essential to keep the affected area clean and dry. Follow these steps when treating jock itch:

- Wash, then dry the area using a clean towel. Use a separate, clean towel on the rest of your body—don't use the same towel you used on your groin.

- Apply the antifungal cream, powder, or spray as directed on the label.

- Change your clothes, especially your underwear, every day.

- Treat other fungal infections, such as athlete's foot.

It's important to continue this treatment for the amount of time recommended in the instructions on the product label. Continue following the steps above even if symptoms disappear sooner to prevent the infection from coming back.

If these steps don't work, or if symptoms last longer than two weeks, talk to your doctor, who might need to prescribe a stronger antifungal cream, spray, or pill.

Can I prevent jock itch?

Good hygiene is the most important thing you can do to help prevent jock itch:

- Shower or take a bath daily, as well as after playing sports.

- Keep the area as dry as possible by always using a clean towel after showering or swimming.

- Avoid sharing towels.

- Wash athletic supporters as often as possible.

If you have a fungal infection somewhere else on your body, like athlete's foot or ringworm, be sure to treat it to help prevent the fungus from spreading to your groin. The best way to prevent the spread is to not touch or scratch your groin area after touching your feet.

Also, use a separate towel on your feet after showering—or if that's not possible, dry your groin before your feet so the towel doesn't spread the infection. If you have athlete's foot, put your socks on before your underwear—this covers your feet so the germs don't get on your underwear.

Jock itch is pretty common. The good news is it can be avoided through proper care and attention—and it's easily treated if you do get it.

Athlete's Foot

What is athlete's foot?

The medical name for athlete's foot is *tinea pedis*. Usually, athlete's foot affects the soles of the feet and the areas between the toes, and it may also spread to the toenails. Athlete's foot can also spread to the palms of your hands, groin, or underarms if you touch your feet and then touch another area of your body.

Athlete's foot doesn't just aggravate athletes; anyone whose feet tend to be damp or sweaty can get this infection. The fungi that cause athlete's foot thrive in warm, moist environments.

The signs and symptoms of athlete's foot include itching, burning, redness, and stinging on the soles of the feet. The skin may flake, peel, blister, or crack.

How can I prevent it?

Athlete's foot is contagious. It's often spread in damp areas, such as public showers or pool areas. To avoid getting athlete's foot, dry your feet—and the spaces between your toes—thoroughly after showering or swimming. Use a clean towel. (Avoid sharing towels because doing so can spread the infection.) If you use public showers, like those in the locker room, wearing waterproof shoes or flip-flops is a good way to protect your feet.

To keep your feet as dry as possible, try not to wear the same shoes or sneakers all the time, and don't wear socks that make your feet sweat or trap moisture. Cotton or wool socks are a good bet. You can also find socks made of special moisture-wicking fabrics in many sports stores—these are designed to keep feet dry.

If possible, choose sneakers that are well ventilated—some sneakers contain small ventilation holes that help to keep your feet dry.

How is athlete's foot treated?

A doctor can often diagnose athlete's foot simply by examining the affected area. Your doctor may also take a small scraping of the skin on your foot. This sample is then examined under a microscope or sent to a laboratory for culture to see if the fungi that cause athlete's foot are present.

If you have athlete's foot, over-the-counter antifungal creams and sprays may solve the problem. Most mild cases of athlete's foot usually clear up within two weeks, but it is common for athlete's foot to recur (come back), so some people use medicated powders and sprays to prevent this from happening.

If an athlete's foot infection is more serious, it can take longer than a couple of weeks to get better. In these cases, it's a good idea to see your doctor, who may prescribe a stronger antifungal cream, spray, or pill.

Chapter 22

Scabies

Scabies is an itchy rash caused by a little mite that burrows in the skin surface. The human scabies mite's scientific name is *Sarcoptes scabiei* var. *hominis*.

How Does One Get Scabies?

Scabies is nearly always acquired by skin-to-skin contact with someone else with scabies. The contact may be quite brief such as holding hands. Frequently it is acquired from children, and sometimes it is sexually transmitted. Occasionally scabies is acquired via bedding or furnishings, as the mite can survive for a few days off its human host.

Scabies is not due to poor hygiene. Nor is it due to animal mites, which do not infest humans. However animal mites can be responsible for bites on exposed sites, usually the forearms.

Typically, an affected host is infested by about 10–12 adult mites. After mating, the male dies. The female scabies mite burrows into the outside layers of the skin where she lays up to three eggs each day for her lifetime of one to two months. The development from egg to adult scabies mite requires 10 to 14 days.

Symptoms And Signs

Itch

The itching appears a few days after infestation. It may occur within a few hours if the mite is caught a second time. The itch is characteristically more severe at night and affects the trunk and limbs. It does not usually affect the scalp.

About This Chapter: "Scabies," reprinted with permission from DermNet NZ, the website of the New Zealand Dermatological Society. Visit www.dermnetnz.org for patient information about skin diseases, conditions, and treatment. © 2013 New Zealand Dermatological Society. All rights reserved.

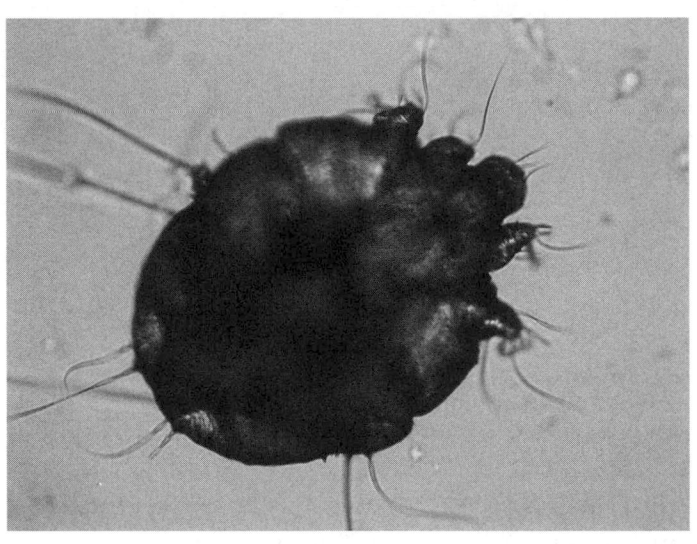

Figure 22.1. Sarcoptes scabiei. (Source: New Zealand Dermatological Society, 2013.)

Burrows

Scabies burrows appear as tiny grey irregular tracks between the fingers and on the wrists. They may also be found in armpits, buttocks, on the penis, insteps, and backs of the heels. Microscopic examination of the contents of a burrow may reveal mites, eggs, or mite feces (scybala).

Generalized Rash

Scabies rash appears as tiny red intensely itchy bumps on the limbs and trunk. It can easily be confused with dermatitis or hives (and may be accompanied by these). The rash of scabies is due to an allergy to the mites and their products and may take several weeks to develop after initial infestation.

Nodules

Itchy lumps or nodules in the armpits and groins or along the shaft of the penis are very suggestive of scabies. Nodules may persist for several weeks or longer after successful eradication of living mite.

Acropustulosis

Blisters and pustules on the palms and soles are characteristic of scabies in infants.

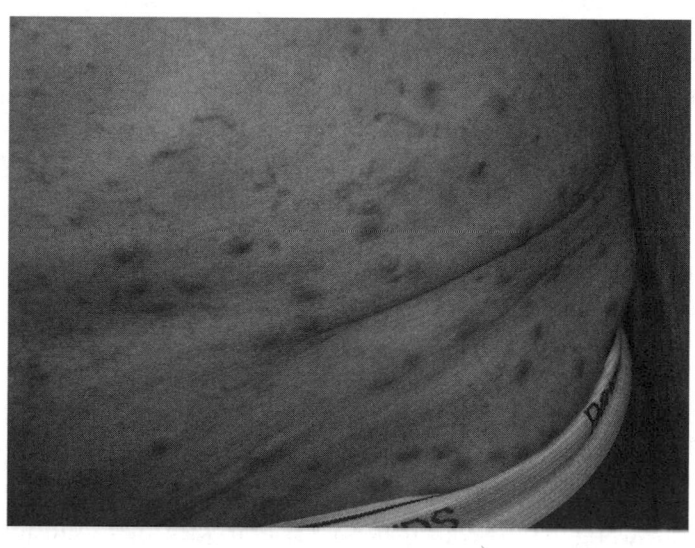

Figure 22.2. Scabetic nodules. (Source: New Zealand Dermatological Society, 2013.)

Secondary Infection

Impetigo commonly complicates scabies and results in crusting patches and scratched pustules. Cellulitis may also occur, resulting in localized painful swelling and redness, associated with fever.

Scabies only rarely affects the face and scalp. This may be the case in young babies and bedbound elderly patients.

Crusted Scabies

Crusted scabies (also called "Norwegian scabies") is a very contagious variant of scabies in which there are thousands or even millions of mites, but very little itch. The patient presents with a generalized scaly rash. It is frequently misdiagnosed as psoriasis. Unlike the usual form of scabies, crusted scabies may affect the scalp.

Crusted scabies is most likely to affect individuals with a poor immune system, neurological diseases, the elderly, or those with mental incompetence. It is the usual cause of severe outbreaks of scabies in an institution such as a hospital, rest home, or prison.

People in contact with someone with crusted scabies may become very itchy, with tiny red spots and blisters on exposed areas; these people are not always infested themselves but must be treated with insecticides just in case they are carrying the mite.

Diagnosis

Scabies can affect children, young adults and the elderly in every community. Think of it if you or your child* has developed a widespread itchy rash, especially if there's been close contact with another itchy person. However, not everyone who itches has scabies; dermatitis is not contagious and is much more common in New Zealand.

If you or your doctor considers scabies a possible explanation for an itchy rash, the diagnosis can be confirmed by microscopic examination of the contents of a burrow. However, even experienced dermatologists only recover a mite or an egg in about 50 percent of cases of scabies.

Occasionally, a skin biopsy is necessary and typical histological features may be seen on pathology.

A new technique using dermoscopy makes it easier to identify a mite at the end of a burrow by its characteristic "jet-plane" appearance.

Treatment

Scabicides are chemical insecticides used to treat scabies. Those available in New Zealand include:

- 25% Benzyl benzoate lotion, applied daily for three days

- 5% Permethrin cream, left on for 8–10 hours

- 0.5% Aqueous malathion lotion, left on for 24 hours

Gamma benzene hexachloride cream is no longer recommended because of resistance and potential toxicity. Sulphur and malathion were popular in the past but are relatively weak scabicides.

The scabicide has to be applied before bed to the whole body from the chin to soles. The scalp and face also need to be treated in children under two years, those confined to bed, and some others with reduced resistance.

A repeat treatment a week later is often recommended. It should not be repeated for several weeks after that without medical advice. Overuse of insecticides will irritate the skin.

Each treatment with scabicide should be followed the next morning by hot-wash laundering or dry cleaning of sheets and pillowcases and any clothes worn against the skin over the last week. Non-washable items should be sealed in a plastic bag and stored above 20° C for one week. Alternatively they can be frozen below -20° C for 12 hours. Rooms should be thoroughly cleaned with normal household products. Fumigation or specialized cleaning is not required. Carpeted floors and upholstered furniture should be vacuumed and all areas cleaned with normal household products. The vacuum bag should then be discarded and furniture covered by plastic or a sheet during treatment and for seven days after.

Most people's itch improves within a few days of treatment but it may take four to six weeks for the itch and rash of scabies to clear completely because of dead mites at the skin surface. These will be slowly cast off.

To reduce the risk of the treatment failing:

- Ensure the scabicide is applied to the whole body from the chin down.

- Leave it on for the recommended time and reapply it after washing.

- Apply the scabicide under fingernails using a soft brush.

- Obtain antibiotics from your doctor if there is crusting and secondary infection.

- Ensure all close contacts are treated whether or not they are itchy.

Persistent Rash

Occasionally a rash persists even though every mite has been killed. Reasons for this include:

- Scabies nodules may take several months to settle down. They are not infectious. A topical steroid may help; apply it accurately to each bump.

- The scabies can result in dermatitis. Dermatitis can be due to the mite, the scratching, the treatment, or other factors. Persistently itchy patches should be treated with frequent applications of emollients and mild topical steroids.

- The diagnosis may be incorrect. Scabies can be confused with a number of other skin conditions, particularly dermatitis and papular urticaria. If you have an itchy rash, your doctor may treat you for scabies 'just in case', even when it is more likely you have another skin disorder. This is because it is important to treat scabies vigorously to prevent other people catching it.

- Resistance to treatment. Scabies occasionally appears to be resistant to the prescribed scabicide. Obtain advice from your doctor; a different scabicide or other treatment may be prescribed. You may be referred to a dermatologist.

Oral ivermectin has proved very effective and is now considered treatment of choice for crusted scabies and other resistant cases.

*Note

Although some of the information in this chapter addresses parents, the facts are also pertinent to teens.

Chapter 23

Swimmer's Itch

What is swimmer's itch?

Swimmer's itch, also called *cercarial dermatitis*, appears as a skin rash caused by an allergic reaction to certain microscopic parasites that infect some birds and mammals. These parasites are released from infected snails into fresh and salt water (such as lakes, ponds, and oceans). While the parasite's preferred host is the specific bird or mammal, if the parasite comes into contact with a swimmer, it burrows into the skin causing an allergic reaction and rash. Swimmer's itch is found throughout the world and is more frequent during summer months.

How does water become infested with the parasite?

The adult parasite lives in the blood of infected animals such as ducks, geese, gulls, swans, and certain mammals such as muskrats and raccoons. The parasites produce eggs that are passed in the feces of infected birds or mammals.

If the eggs land in or are washed into the water, the eggs hatch, releasing small, free-swimming microscopic larvae. These larvae swim in the water in search of a certain species of aquatic snail.

If the larvae find one of these snails, they infect the snail, multiply and undergo further development. Infected snails release a different type of microscopic larvae (or *cercariae*, hence the name *cercarial dermatitis*) into the water. This larval form then swims about searching for a suitable host (bird, muskrat) to continue the lifecycle. Although humans are not suitable hosts, the microscopic larvae burrow into the swimmer's skin, and may cause an allergic reaction and rash. Because these larvae cannot develop inside a human, they soon die.

About This Chapter: Text in this chapter is from "Swimmer's Itch FAQs," Centers for Disease Control and Prevention (www.cdc.gov), January 10, 2012.

What are the signs and symptoms of swimmer's itch?

Symptoms of swimmer's itch may include the following:

- Tingling, burning, or itching of the skin

- Small reddish pimples

- Small blisters

Within minutes to days after swimming in contaminated water, you may experience tingling, burning, or itching of the skin. Small reddish pimples appear within 12 hours. Pimples may develop into small blisters. Scratching the areas may result in secondary bacterial infections. Itching may last up to a week or more, but will gradually go away.

Because swimmer's itch is caused by an allergic reaction to infection, the more often you swim or wade in contaminated water, the more likely you are to develop more serious symptoms. The greater the number of exposures to contaminated water, the more intense and immediate symptoms of swimmer's itch will be.

Be aware that swimmer's itch is not the only rash that may occur after swimming in fresh or salt water.

Do I need to see my health care provider for treatment?

Most cases of swimmer's itch do not require medical attention. If you have a rash, you may try the following for relief:

- Use corticosteroid cream.

- Apply cool compresses to the affected areas.

- Bathe in Epsom salts or baking soda.

- Soak in colloidal oatmeal baths.

- Apply baking soda paste to the rash (made by stirring water into baking soda until it reaches a paste-like consistency).

- Use an anti-itch lotion.

Though difficult, try not to scratch. Scratching may cause the rash to become infected. If itching is severe, your health care provider may suggest prescription-strength lotions or creams to lessen your symptoms.

Can swimmer's itch be spread from person-to-person?

Swimmer's itch is not contagious and cannot be spread from one person to another.

Who is at risk for swimmer's itch?

Anyone who swims or wades in infested water may be at risk. Larvae are more likely to be present in shallow water by the shoreline. Children are most often affected because they tend to swim, wade, and play in the shallow water more than adults. Also, they are less likely to towel dry themselves when leaving the water.

Once an outbreak of swimmer's itch has occurred in water, will the water always be unsafe?

No. Many factors must be present for swimmer's itch to become a problem in water. Since these factors change (sometimes within a swim season), swimmer's itch will not always be a problem. However, there is no way to know how long water may be unsafe. Larvae generally survive for 24 hours once they are released from the snail. However, an infected snail will continue to produce *cercariae* throughout the remainder of its life. For future snails to become infected, migratory birds or mammals in the area must also be infected so the lifecycle can continue.

Is it safe to swim in my swimming pool?

Yes. As long as your swimming pool is well maintained and chlorinated, there is no risk of swimmer's itch. The appropriate snails must be present in order for swimmer's itch to occur.

What can be done to reduce the risk of swimmer's itch?

To reduce the likelihood of developing swimmer's itch, follow these guidelines:

- Do not swim in areas where swimmer's itch is a known problem or where signs have been posted warning of unsafe water.

- Do not swim near or wade in marshy areas where snails are commonly found.

- Towel dry or shower immediately after leaving the water. Do not attract birds (for example, by feeding them) to areas where people are swimming.

- Encourage health officials to post signs on shorelines where swimmer's itch is a current problem.

Part Four
Other Diseases And Disorders Affecting The Skin

Chapter 24

Birthmarks

About Birthmarks

A birthmark is a skin marking which is present at birth or appears shortly after birth, usually within the first two months of life. Dermatologists divide birthmarks into two main categories—vascular "red" birthmarks and pigmented birthmarks.

What are vascular "red" birthmarks?

Red birthmarks are a caused by an overgrowth of blood vessels.

What are some common types of vascular "red" birthmarks?

There are many different kinds of vascular birthmarks, but the three most common types are macular stains, hemangiomas, and port wine stains. The different types of birthmarks have their own appearance and typical locations that are usually affected. Brief descriptions of these common types are discussed below.

Macular Stains

Also called "salmon patches," this is the most common type of vascular birthmark. They are faint, mild red or pink in color, and flat. They are commonly called "angel's kisses" when they are located on the forehead, eyelids, tip of the nose, or upper lip or "stork bites" on the back of the neck. Stork bites appear on 30 to 50 percent of newborn babies and usually persist into adulthood, but are often covered by hair once it grows in as the child ages. Angel's kisses most often fade as the infant grows and will go away by age two.

Hemangiomas

Hemangiomas are usually divided into two types based on how extensive the development of blood vessels at the site is underneath the skin: Superficial hemangiomas (strawberry hemangiomas, strawberry mark, nevus vascularis, capillary hemangioma, hemangioma simplex) and deep hemangiomas (cavernous hemangioma, angioma cavernosum, cavernoma). Superficial hemangiomas tend to be raised and bright red in color because the abnormal blood vessels are very close to the surface of the skin, whereas deep hemangiomas tend to be bluish-purple in color because the abnormal blood vessels are deeper under the skin. They might be absent at birth, and develop after several weeks and are more common in females, multiple gestations like twins, and premature babies. Usually a baby will have only one hemangioma, but in very rare cases, an infant may have many or even some internally. Unlike the other types of vascular birthmarks, hemangiomas typically grow very rapidly for several months, then they become white-grey in color and slowly shrink in most cases. Fifty percent of all hemangiomas are flat by age five and about 90 percent are flat by age nine. It is impossible to predict how big any hemangioma will grow, or if it will completely disappear. Some slight discoloration or puckering of the skin might remain at the site of the hemangioma.

Port-Wine Stains

Port-wine stains are flat, purple-to-red birthmarks made of dilated blood capillaries that appear at birth. These birthmarks occur most often on the face and might vary in size. Port-wine stains often are permanent (unless treated) and might thicken, develop small bumps or ridges, or darken over time. Rarely, port-wine stains on the forehead, eyes, or both sides of the face can be associated with glaucoma and/or seizures and those children should be evaluated by a physician to monitor for those complications.

What are the symptoms of red birthmarks?

Symptoms of red birthmarks include:

- Skin markings that develop before or shortly after birth
- Red skin rashes or lesions—may be more noticeable when the infant cries or during temperature changes
- Itching
- Open sore or ulcer
- Possible bleeding

How are red birthmarks diagnosed?

In most cases, a health care professional can diagnose a red birthmark based on the appearance of the skin. Deeper birthmarks can be confirmed with imaging tests such as MRI, ultrasound, CT scans, or biopsies.

What is the treatment for red birthmarks?

Birthmarks rarely cause problems, other than cosmetic changes. Many birthmarks are temporary and will go away on their own by the time a child is of school age; however some are permanent. Permanent birthmarks are usually not treated unless they cause unwanted symptoms, or until a child is at least school age. Some indications for treating red birthmarks are disfiguring appearance, psychological distress, pain, bleeding, rapid increase in size, and at-risk locations such as the eye where it may obstruct vision or near other vital structures.

Some treatment methods for red birthmarks include:

- Concealing cosmetics
- Topical or injected corticosteroids
- Topical or oral beta blockers
- Cryotherapy (freezing)
- Laser surgery
- Surgical removal

Can red birthmarks be prevented?

Currently, there is no known way to prevent red birthmarks.

What are pigmented birthmarks?

Pigmented birthmarks are areas in which the color of the birthmark is different from the color of the rest of the skin. The marks range in color from tan, brown, black, blue, or blue-gray.

What are the types of pigmented birthmarks?

Mongolian spots are usually are bluish and look like bruises. They often appear on the buttocks and/or lower back, but they sometimes also appear on the trunk or arms. These spots are seen most often in people who have darker skin.

Congenital nevi are moles that are present at birth. About 1 in 100 people are born with one or more moles. These birthmarks have a slightly increased risk of becoming skin cancer, depending on their size. Larger congenital nevi (>20 cm) have a greater risk of developing into skin cancer than do smaller congenital nevi. All congenital nevi should be examined by a health care provider, and any change in the birthmark should be reported.

Cafe-au-lait spots are light tan or light brown spots that are usually oval in shape. They usually appear at birth but might develop in the first few years of a child's life. Cafe-au-lait spots might be a normal type of birthmark, but the presence of several cafe-au-lait spots larger than a quarter might occur in neurofibromatosis (a genetic disorder that causes abnormal cell growth of nerve tissues) and other conditions.

What causes pigmented birthmarks?

The cause of pigmented birthmarks is not known.

What are the symptoms of pigmented birthmarks?

Pigmented birthmarks might increase in size as the child grows, change colors (especially after sun exposure and during the teen years as hormone levels change), become itchy, and might occasionally bleed.

How are pigmented birthmarks diagnosed?

In most cases, health care professionals can diagnose birthmarks based on the appearance of the skin. If needed, a skin biopsy might be performed.

How are pigmented birthmarks treated?

In most cases, no treatment is needed for pigmented birthmarks. When birthmarks do require treatment, however, that treatment varies based on the age of the child, the type of birthmark and its related conditions, and its location. Typically surgical excision is the indicated treatment in these cases.

What are the complications of pigmented birthmarks?

Some complications of pigmented birthmarks can include psychological effects in cases in which the birthmark is prominent. Pigmented birthmarks also can pose an increased skin cancer risk.

A doctor should check any changes that occur in the color, size, or texture of a nevus or other skin lesion. See a doctor right away if there is any pain, bleeding, itching, inflammation, or ulceration of a congenital nevus or other skin lesion.

Can pigmented birthmarks be prevented?

There is no known way to prevent birthmarks. People with birthmarks should use a good-quality sunscreen when outdoors in order to prevent complications.

Chapter 25

Cellulite And Stretch Marks

Cellulite

Cellulite is fat that is deposited in pockets just below the surface of the skin. It occurs around the hips, thighs, and buttocks. Because it is very close to the surface of the skin, cellulite leads to a dimpled appearance.

Information

Cellulite may be more visible than fat deeper in the body. Even thin people can have cellulite, because we all have layers of fat just below the surface of the skin. Collagen fibers that connect fat to the skin may stretch, break down, or pull tight, allowing the fat cells to bulge out. This creates the rippled look of cellulite.

Your genes may play a part in whether or not you have cellulite. A poor diet, "fad" dieting, a slow metabolism, hormone changes, and even dehydration may play a role. A great deal of money is spent by people who want to rid themselves of cellulite, but no amount of weight loss, exercise, massages, wraps, creams, supplements, or surgery has proven to effectively eliminate it once you have it. Liposuction, for instance, is not recommended for cellulite, and may even make it look worse.

Although many dermatologists and cosmetic surgeons recognize cellulite as a legitimate problem that patients seek to have them "cure," most of the medical community doesn't view cellulite as a disorder. Instead, it is considered a normal condition of many women and some men.

About This Chapter: From "Cellulite" and "Striae," © 2013 A.D.A.M., Inc. Reprinted with permission.

Tips for avoiding cellulite include:

- Eating a healthy diet rich in fruits, vegetables, and fiber
- Staying hydrated with plenty of fluids
- Exercising regularly to keep muscles toned and bones strong
- Maintaining a healthy weight (no yo-yo dieting)
- Not smoking

Striae

Striae are irregular areas of skin that look like bands, stripes, or lines. Striae are seen when a person grows or gains weight rapidly or has certain diseases or conditions.

Striae are commonly called stretch marks.

Considerations

Stretch marks can appear when there is rapid stretching of the skin. They are often associated with the abdominal enlargement of pregnancy. They can be found in children who have become rapidly obese. They may also occur during the rapid growth of puberty in males and females. Striae are most commonly located on the breasts, hips, thighs, buttocks, abdomen, and flank.

Stretch marks appear as parallel streaks of red, thinned, glossy skin that over time become whitish and scarlike in appearance. The stretch marks may be slightly depressed and have a different texture than normal skin.

Striae may also occur as a result of abnormal collagen formation, or a result of medications or chemicals that interfere with collagen formation. They may also be associated with longtime use of cortisone compounds, diabetes, Cushing disease, and post-pregnancy.

Causes

- Cushing syndrome
- Ehlers-Danlos syndrome
- Pregnancy
- Puberty
- Obesity
- Overuse of cortisone skin creams

Home Care

There is no specific care for stretch marks. Marks often will disappear after the cause of the skin stretching is gone. Creams and ointments that claim to prevent stretch marks during pregnancy are of little value.

Avoiding rapid weight gain helps reduce stretch marks caused by obesity.

When To Contact A Medical Professional

If striae or stretch marks appear without obvious cause such as pregnancy or rapid weight gain, call your health care provider.

What To Expect At Your Office Visit

You health care provider will examine you and ask questions about your symptoms, including:

- Is this the first time that you have developed striae?

- When did you first notice the stretch marks?

- What medicines have you taken?

- Have you used a cortisone skin cream?

- What other symptoms do you have?

If the striae are not caused by normal physical changes, tests may be done. Topical retinoids can be prescribed and may help the appearance of striae. Laser treatment may also help. However, striae are difficult to treat.

Alternative Names

Striae atrophica; Stretch marks; Striae distensae

Chapter 26

Cysts: Epidermoid (Sebaceous), Pilonidal, And Lipoma

Cyst

A cyst is a closed pocket or pouch of tissue. It can be filled with air, fluid, pus, or other material.

Considerations

Cysts may form within any tissue in the body. Cysts within the lung generally are air-filled, while cysts involving the lymph system or kidneys are fluid-filled. Certain parasites, such as trichinosis, dog tapeworm (*Toxocara canis*), and echinococcus, can form cysts within the muscles, liver, brain, lungs, and eyes.

Cysts are common on the skin. They develop as a result of infection, clogging of sebaceous glands (acne-related cysts), or around a foreign object stuck in the skin.

Sebaceous Cyst

A sebaceous cyst is a closed sac under the skin filled with a cheese-like or oily material.

Causes

Sebaceous cysts most often arise from swollen hair follicles. Skin trauma can also induce a cyst to form. A sac of cells is created into which a protein called keratin is secreted.

These cysts are usually found on the face, neck, and trunk. They are usually slow-growing, painless, freely movable lumps beneath the skin. Occasionally, however, a cyst will become inflamed and tender.

Symptoms

The main symptom is usually a small, non-painful lump beneath the skin. If the lump becomes infected or inflamed, other symptoms may include:

- Skin redness
- Tender or sore skin
- Warm skin in the affected area

Grayish-white, cheesy, foul-smelling material may drain from the cyst.

Exams And Tests

In most cases, your doctor can diagnose this type of cyst by simply examining your skin. Occasionally, a biopsy may be needed to rule out other conditions.

Treatment

Sebaceous cysts are not dangerous and can usually be ignored. Placing a warm moist cloth (compress) over the area may help the cyst drain and heal.

If you have a small inflamed cyst, your doctor may inject it with a steroid medicine that reduces swelling.

If the cyst becomes swollen, tender, or large, your doctor may drain it or perform surgery to remove it.

Outlook (Prognosis)

Large, painful cysts may interfere with day-to-day life.

Possible Complications

These cysts may occasionally become infected and form painful abscesses.

The cysts may return after they are surgically removed.

When To Contact A Medical Professional

Call your health care provider if you notice any new growths on your body. Although cysts are not dangerous, your doctor should examine you for signs of skin cancer.

Alternative Names

Epidermal cyst; Keratin cyst; Epidermoid cyst

Pilonidal Dimple

Pilonidal dimple is a condition that can occur anywhere along the crease between the buttocks, which runs from the bone at the bottom of the spine (sacrum) to the anus.

Pilonidal dimple may appear as:

- A pilonidal abscess, in which the hair follicle becomes infected and pus collects in the fat tissue

- A pilonidal cyst, in which a cyst or hole forms if there has been an abscess for a long time

- A pilonidal sinus, in which a tract grows under the skin or deeper from the hair follicle

- A small pit or pore in the skin that contains dark spots or hair

Considerations

Symptoms may include:

- Pus may drain to a small pit in the skin
- Tenderness over the area after you are active or sit for a period of time
- Warm, tender, swollen area near the tailbone
- Fever (rare)

There may be no symptoms other than a small dent (pit) in the skin in the crease between the buttocks.

Causes

The cause of pilonidal disease is not clear. It is thought to be caused by hair growing into the skin in the crease between the buttocks.

This problem is more likely to occur in people who:

- Are obese
- Experienced trauma or irritation in the area
- Have excess body hair
- Sit for long periods of time
- Wear tight clothing

145

Home Care

It may help to keep the area clean and dry and remove hair regularly to prevent infection.

When To Contact A Medical Professional

Call your health care provider if you notice any of the following around the pilonidal cyst:

- Drainage of pus
- Redness
- Swelling
- Tenderness

Lipoma

A lipoma is a soft, fatty lump that grows under the skin. It is harmless and can usually be left alone.

Lipomas can occur on any area of skin where there are fat cells, but are usually seen on the shoulders, neck, chest, arms, and back. They range from the size of a pea to a few centimeters across and grow very slowly.

About 1 in 100 people develop a lipoma, so they are fairly common. It is unusual to develop more than one or two lipomas, unless you have a rare inherited condition called familial multiple lipomatosis, which causes lipomas to develop all over the body.

Lipoma Or Cyst?

A cyst is a sac under the skin that contains fluid (usually pus) and can look a bit like a lipoma. Here's how to tell the difference:

- Cysts are close to the skin surface, whereas lipomas are deeper under the skin.
- Cysts are firm to the touch; lipomas are soft and dough-like.
- The skin may be inflamed (red and swollen) with a cyst, but not with a lipoma.

When To See Your Doctor

You can usually tell if a bump is a lipoma by pressing it. It should feel smooth and soft, like rubber or dough, and may move about under the skin.

If you are unsure whether it is a lipoma or you are worried it could be more serious, see your doctor. They can usually confirm whether the lump is a lipoma just by examining it. If there is any doubt about the diagnosis, the lipoma may be removed.

What To Expect At Your Office Visit

You will be asked for your medical history and given a physical examination. Sometimes you may be asked for the following information:

- Has there been any change in the appearance of the pilonidal cyst?

- Has there been any drainage from the area?

- Do you have any other symptoms?

Rarely, a CT scan is done.

Pilonidal disease that causes no symptoms does not need to be treated.

A lipoma is just a collection of fat cells and there is no evidence it will turn into skin cancer.

Also see your doctor if your lump:

- Changes in any way
- Grows back after it has been removed
- Feels hard
- Is painful

In this case, your doctor will want to rule out either angiolipoma, a benign lipoma caused by an increase in small blood vessels, or liposarcoma, a very rare type of soft tissue cancer.

Getting A Lipoma Removed

You may want your lipoma removed if it's large or in an obvious place and affecting your self-esteem.

A lipoma may also need to be removed if it is causing discomfort. For example, it may be pressing on a nerve and causing pain.

Some privately practicing doctors will be able to remove lipomas. Otherwise, you will need to have this procedure done in hospital as a day patient (you do not need to stay overnight).

You will be given an injection of local anesthetic, which will numb the area, before the doctor cuts the skin over the bump and removes the lipoma. The wound will be closed with stitches and you will be left with a fine scar.

Source: "Lipoma," reprinted from NHS Choices, www.nhs.uk. Reproduced by kind permission of the Department of Health, © 2013.

A pilonidal abscess may be opened, drained, and packed with gauze. Antibiotics may be used if there is an infection spreading in the skin or you also have another, more severe illness.

Other surgeries that may be needed include:

- Removal (excision) of the diseased area

- Skin grafts

- Surgery to remove an abscess that returns

Alternative Names

Pilonidal abscess; Pilonidal sinus; Pilonidal cyst; Pilonidal disease

Chapter 27

Eczema (Atopic Dermatitis)

Eczema, also called **atopic dermatitis**, is a chronic skin that causes areas of red, itchy skin. This condition usually starts in early childhood, especially when there is a family history of atopy (asthma, hay fever, conjunctivitis, or food allergies). The skin fails to hold in moisture, becomes dry, then inflamed, itchy, and often infected. Various combinations of factors cause the dryness. Allergies leading to an overactive immune system and hereditary dry skin (ichthyosis vulgaris) are the most prominent internal and external factors.

To treat this disease you need to work with the doctor in identifying and reducing those factors in your or your child's life that trigger of flare-up the disease. These are different for each person, so no one therapy is appropriate for all eczema patients. You need to watch for some of the following possible exacerbating factors.

Eczema: Irritants

Environmental factors can have a big effect on your eczema. To prevent irritation, you should minimize the use of soaps. Deodorant soaps are often very harsh and drying. If you need them, limit their use to areas that develop an odor such as the armpits, genital area, and feet. Recommended soaps are Dove, Olay, and Basis. Even better than soap is non-soap cleansing agents such as Cetaphil Lotion, Oilatum-AD, and Aquanil. Since residual laundry detergent in clothes may also be irritating, in some a second rinse cycle is beneficial. Use a perfume and color free detergent such as Cheer Free or All Free.

Hand dermatitis occurs commonly in adult eczema patients. Here it is especially important to avoid irritant contact with solvents, soaps, and detergents. Also avoid jobs and hobbies that require exposure to these irritants, as well as to dust, dirt, and heat. If you wash frequently, it is important to apply moisturizers after hand washing; also trying a non-water cleansing method, such as Cetaphil, may be beneficial. Wearing appropriate gloves when using potential irritants is also important. There are barrier creams, which can be applied 10–15 minutes before coming into contact with irritants, that may help reduce flares.

If sweating causes itching, modify your activity and surroundings to minimize sweating. Work and sleep in a fairly constant temperature (68–75° F) and humidity (45–55%). Wear open-weave, loose-fitting garments made of cotton blends, rather than wool or stiff fabrics.

Eczema: Allergens

Allergens in the air and in the food are often triggers for a flare-up of this disorder. If you can furnish a list on how your disease gets activated, the doctor may try to correlate this with a skin (prick or intradermal) or blood (RAST) test. Don't try to avoid everything that might be considered an allergen without any incriminating evidence. Occasionally, using an air purifier can help reduce allergen exposure at home or in the workplace.

Dust mite allergy is the most important home allergen. Go after the dust mites; almost all atopics are highly sensitive to dust mites. There are dust mite covers to enclose mattresses and box springs. Try Vellux blankets. You may need a dehumidifier to keep relative humidity below 50% since mites thrive in humid environments and an acaracide such as benzyl benzoate (Acarosan) to carpeting. Removal of fitted carpets in the bedroom should be recommended. Get new pillows and wash the duvets and pillows every three months; washes should be hotter than 55° C to kill mites and denature antigens. Reducing upholstered furnishings and regular use of a modern cylinder or upright vacuum cleaner fitted with an adequate filter.

Infantile eczema is often allergy related in the first year of life. Peanuts, wheat, soy, whole milk, eggs, and citrus are the common offenders. Great care is needed if the diet is changed because malnutrition can do more harm in the long run than eczema. Lamb, chicken, and rice are usually completely safe. Breast milk is the best "formula," and then try soy formulas. If there is no improvement consider goat's milk. Allergy tests (both skin and blood) are not completely reliable for foods, but may at times be helpful. Eliminate a suspected food, but if no clear benefit is obtained after four weeks, do not continue.

As the child grows, many food allergies often fade or disappear. In the small minority of eczema sufferers who get real benefit from food avoidance there is great benefit. Care must be taken to avoid malnutrition when any restrictive diets are used. In small children special diets are difficult to implement, and the help of a dietitian is necessary.

There are studies showing breast-feeding may delay the onset of eczema if practiced for at least the first three to six months of life. Some mothers also avoid cows milk and other possible food allergens during pregnancy and nursing, but this is unproven.

Eczema: Infections

Flare-ups and hard to control eczema are often due to a coexisting bacterial, and sometimes fungus or virus, infection. If your eczema is weeping or oozing, if it crusted, or if it has small bumps, your doctor will probably test or treat for bacterial infection.

Systemic antibiotics are often necessary to decrease the irritation caused by *Staph* bacteria on the skin. Most patients with eczema have *Staph* bacteria on their skin, and this can cause irritation even without overt infection. In acute flares, antibiotic treatment usually lasts from 14 to 28 days. Chronic maintenance antibiotics may be used if you develop infections repeatedly. Some have found success by adding very dilute bleach to the bathwater—no more than a tablespoon for a full bathtub. Topical antibiotics like Neosporin should not be recommended and most antibacterial cleansers may worsen the condition.

Rarely, the cold sore virus (*Herpes simplex*) may cause extensive local or widespread infection, and is usually treated with oral antiviral medication.

Treatment

Your skin is dry, not because it lacks grease or oil, but because it fails to retain water. Therefore, to correct dryness, water is added to the skin, followed by a grease or oil-containing substance to hold the water in.

Soaking the affected area, in a basin, bath, or shower, for 15–20 minutes using lukewarm water, can help to hydrate the skin. Hot water dries out the skin. Then, remove excess water by patting with a soft towel. Avoid vigorous use of a washcloth in cleansing. When toweling dry, do not rub the skin. Blot or pat dry so there is still some moisture left on the skin, and immediately apply a moisturizing cream (Eucerin Cream, Moisturel Cream, Cetaphil Cream). Moisturizing lotions contain some water, so they do not work as well. Use of moisturizers without first trapping in water is much less effective. Many patients find that two or three additional applications of moisturizers during the day give additional help.

Tar Preparations

Tars and extracts of crude coal tar are often used to reduce the amount of topical steroids needed in chronic maintenance of eczema. A pharmacist can make up 1% to 5% percent LCD (liquor carbonis detergens) in a cream. Tar gel products (Estar Gel and Psorigel) are available, but they contain alcohol and may cause burning and irritation on already red and inflamed skin.

Steroids

Topical steroids are particularly useful to treat flare-ups of eczema. They help keep down the inflammation and itching. Apply them just on the rash (instead of the oil recommended above) especially after a soak or bath. Do not use topical steroids more than twice a day. Your pharmacist can provide topical steroids in large jars to reduce the cost.

Hydrocortisone ointment or cream can be used for eczema in infants and young children, or in skin folds in adults. More potent topical steroids should not be used on thin-skinned areas of the face, neck, axilla, and groin. Short, supervised courses of medium potency topical steroids creams are safe and effective for flares of eczema on other parts of the body. Adverse effects of long-term topical steroids include thinning of the skin (atrophy), a change in the color of some skin (depigmentation), and acne-like eruptions.

A newer class of topical drugs are the "topical immunomodulators" or TIMs. These locally calm down the immune system similar to topical steroids. However they don't have the side effect of steroids in that they do not cause thinning of the skin with long-term use. There are currently two of these drugs available: Protopic (tacrolimus) Ointment and Elidel (pimecrolimus) Cream. They can be used in patients two years of age or older.

Ultraviolet Light

Ultraviolet light (UVB or PUVA) therapy may be of some help in chronic eczema that does not respond well to other therapy. UVB and PUVA require three per week and must be used under professional supervision. However, avoid sunburn and hot or humid conditions that might make your skin even itchier. The risks of UVB or PUVA are sunburn and increased risk of skin cancers if used for too long.

Antipruritics

Itching is often the most aggravating of all your eczema symptoms. Antihistamines may provide some relief. The antihistamines reduce scratching mainly through tranquilizing and sedative effects. It takes several weeks of use on a regular basis to help. This is because scratching aggravates the eczema, keeping it from healing. Cutting nails and using cotton gloves at night can minimize scratching. For children, knee-high socks are better than gloves, because they are harder to accidentally pull off during sleep. The topical use of antihistamines such as Benadryl should be avoided, because it is ineffective and may produce allergic reactions. Menthol- or pramoxine-containing products such as Aveeno cream, Pramasone cream/lotion or Prax lotion may offer additional help.

Evolving Treatments

Recently treatments with drugs that work on a system that is related to the one aspirin works on have been used for asthma. These medications have few side effects (an occasional headache mostly) and show good result in a little under half the people treated. Adults are usually given Accolate (zafirlukast) 20 milligrams (mg) twice daily, children over six years get Singulair (montelukast) 5 mg chewable daily and younger get one-half of a 5 mg chewable tab per day. About a third of the most severe eczema patients will improve with the drug hydroxychloroquine. All will clear completely within weeks if given, but long term damage to the kidneys prevents its use except for short periods.

Corticosteroids

Oral steroids should be minimized because of the seriousness of their side effects and the potential for severe flares of eczema when they are discontinued. If these are used for severe flares, then intensified skin care will help to suppress the flaring of the eczema during a taper from oral steroids.

Therapy Of Acute Flares

The doctor may suggest hospitalization simply because it may be necessary to break the cycle of chronic inflammation, or other problems that are exacerbating the illness. Frequently, five or six days of vigorous in-hospital treatment care can result in a dramatic clearing of the eczema. Food tests, allergy skin testing, and the development of an outpatient therapy plan can all be done during the hospitalization. Unfortunately, getting approval from insurers is often difficult. During an acute flare the number of 15–20 minute baths must be increased to three or four per day. Besides hydrating the skin, baths also increase the penetration of topical medication up to 10-fold if the medicine is applied immediately after the bath. Wet wraps after baths may also help hydration and medicinal penetration. Bedtime wet wraps are most practical, and can be done with elasticized gauze followed by ace bandages or double pajamas. (The first pair of pajamas is worn damp but not soaking wet, and a second pair of dry pajamas is worn over them. For a tighter fit, sometimes a plastic sauna suit is used instead of the dry pajamas.) For feet and hands, socks can be used. Additional blankets or increased room heat may be necessary during this three to seven days to prevent chilling.

Chapter 28

Hyperhidrosis (Excessive Sweating)

Hyperhidrosis is the medical term for **excessive sweating**. The problem may be limited to a few problem areas or may be all over. The armpits and the palms are the areas most often troublesome. Excessive sweating starts after puberty. It may be present to some degree all the time, but is at its worst when under stress such as during exams, interviews, or dating. Excess sweating that affects areas other than the armpits and palms may a sign of serious problems. Systemic, neurological, and anxiety conditions need to be ruled out; however most cases have no underlying cause.

Most over-the-counter antiperspirants are not strong enough to do the job. The best topical product, Drysol, is available by prescription. It may be somewhat irritating and sometimes takes a while to get used to it. Drysol is applied at bedtime to completely dry skin and washed off in the morning shower. Do not use a regular deodorant afterwards. Repeat the treatment nightly until the sweating is under control. If it does not work after one or two weeks, begin covering the affected area with a square of "Saran Wrap" overnight. After it begins to work, use once or twice weekly to maintain the effect, and use a regular deodorant on the other days. The medication is less effective on the thick skin of the palms and soles.

If this treatment doesn't work well enough there are alternatives. Botox injections, a treatment popular for wrinkles, will control excessive sweating for four to six months. Botox is a purified protein which has the ability to block the chemical which activates sweat glands. The U.S. Food and Drug Administration (FDA) has approved this treatment for underarm hyperhidrosis. Many insurances are now covering the cost of Botox for this condition. Some physicians are using Botox for sweating of the palms, however sometimes it may cause a temporary weakness of the grip.

Another treatment option is iontophoresis. This is especially good for palmar sweating in people who do not respond well to topical products. Iontophoresis uses an electrical device connected to a water bath. Hands are placed in the bath and a weak electrical current is conducted through the skin which inhibits sweating. There are no significant side effects from long-term use of this device. For mild hyperhidrosis, the battery powered Drionic device may be helpful, and can be purchased without a prescription. A stronger option is the plug in iontophoresis unit, which does need a prescription. In the U.S., it may be rented or purchased from the R.A. Fischer Company.

People who have not had success with the above treatments may consider oral medications, including Robinul and Pro-Banthine pills. This is an especially good option when someone has generalized sweating. These drugs are fairly safe but may have some annoying side effects including dry mouth, constipation, urine retention, blurring of vision, and heart palpitations. Since these side effects are dose dependent, it's best to start with a low dose and slowly increase the dose if needed.

A surgical procedure called "endoscopic thoracic sympathectomy" can cure hyperhidrosis of the palms. An experienced surgeon must do it. It may cause some increased sweating on other parts of the body, but most patients don't seem to be bothered by this. Some liposuction surgeons know a special technique to scrape out the sweat glands from the armpits. These treatments should be discussed in detail before they are considered.

The newest treatment for hyperhidrosis is miraDry. It was approved by the FDA in 2011 for excessive underarm sweating. This treatment uses a hand held device which delivers electromagnetic energy non-invasively to the area where the sweat glands reside. As a result the glands are destroyed and don't grow back, resulting in a dramatic and lasting reduction of underarm sweat.

The International Hyperhidrosis Society's website (www.sweathelp.org) contains more information about these treatments.

Chapter 29

Keloids

The body's tissue naturally heals itself when it is damaged. This healing process can cause scars to appear.

If the skin is broken (for example by a cut, bite, scratch, burn, or acne), the body produces more of a protein called collagen.

What are keloid scars?

Collagen gathers around the damage and builds up to help the wound seal over. The resulting scar usually fades over time, becoming smoother and less noticeable. However, some scars don't stop growing. They "invade" the surrounding healthy skin and become bigger than the original wound. These are known as keloid scars.

"A keloid scar is an overgrown scar that can spread outside the original area of skin damage," says Indy Rihal of the British Skin Foundation. "Keloid scars are shiny and hairless, they're raised above the surrounding skin, and can feel hard and rubbery." Keloids affect around 10–15 percent of all wounds. They can appear anywhere on the body but usually form on the shoulders, head, and neck.

They can last for years and sometimes don't form until months or years after the initial injury. New keloid scars are sometimes red or purple. They're not usually painful, but some people feel embarrassed or upset if they think the scar is disfiguring them.

Experts don't fully understand why keloid scarring happens, but these scars are not contagious (they're not catching) and there is no risk of them turning into cancer.

About This Chapter: "Keloid Scarring," reprinted from NHS Choices, www.nhs.uk. Reproduced by kind permission of the Department of Health, © 2013.

Who gets keloid scars?

"People with dark skin get keloids much more easily than people with fairer skin, and it's common in people with black skin," says Rihal. "They're most common between the ages of 10 and 30, and can run in families."

Keloid scars can develop after even a very minor injury. "Burns, acne scars, and wounds that get infected are particularly likely to form keloids," says Rihal. "You're at higher risk of getting a keloid scar if you have had one before."

Can I reduce the risk?

You can't stop a keloid from happening, but you can avoid any deliberate cuts or breaks in the skin, such as tattoos or piercings, including on the earlobes.

What is the treatment for keloid scars?

There are several treatments available, but none of them has been shown to be more effective than the others. Treatment can be difficult and isn't always successful. Treatments that may help flatten a keloid include:

- Steroid injections

- Applying steroid-impregnated tape to the area for 12 hours a day

- Applying a silicone sheet to the area at night for several months (however, there is not much evidence that this works)

Other options are:

- Freezing early keloids with liquid nitrogen to stop them from growing

- Laser treatment to lessen redness (this won't make the scar any smaller)

- Surgery to remove the keloid (however, the keloid can grow back and may be larger than before)

If you're bothered by a keloid scar and want help, see your family doctor.

Chapter 30

Lichen Sclerosus

What Is Lichen Sclerosus?

Lichen sclerosus is chronic skin disorder that most often affects the genital and perianal areas. It usually persists for years, and can cause permanent scarring. There is no known cure, although most people are substantially improved and quite comfortable with treatment. The condition was previously known as "lichen sclerosus et atrophicus."

Lichen sclerosus (LS) is 10 times more common in women than in men. It can start at any age, although it is most often seen in women over 50. Prepubertal girls can also be affected. It may cause no symptoms but it can be itchy, sometimes severely so. It can develop after an injury to the affected area. It may follow or co-exist with another skin condition such as lichen simplex, candidiasis, or erosive lichen planus.

What Does It Look Like?

Lichen sclerosus presents as white crinkled or thickened patches.

Vulval Lichen Sclerosus

In women, lichen sclerosus results in a white thickening of the skin of the vulva. It can be localized to one small area or involving the perineum, labia majora, labia minora, fourchette, and clitoris. Sometimes the clitoris disappears, the labia (lips) can shrink and the entrance to the vagina tightens. Lichen sclerosus never affects inside the vagina.

About This Chapter: "Lichen Sclerosus," reprinted with permission from DermNet NZ, the website of the New Zealand Dermatological Society. Visit www.dermnetnz.org for patient information about skin diseases, conditions, and treatment. © 2013 New Zealand Dermatological Society. All rights reserved.

The affected skin can be unbearably itchy (the symptom known as pruritus vulvae) and/or sore (vulvodynia). Sometimes bruises, blood blisters, and ulcers appear, after scratching, or on their own.

Sexual intercourse can be very uncomfortable and may result in splitting of the skin (fissuring).

The skin around the anus may be affected by lichen sclerosus, which may cause discomfort or bleeding when passing bowel motions, and aggravate any tendency to constipation particularly in children.

Lichen sclerosus is associated with an increased risk of vulvar cancer, which presents as a slowly growing lump or a sore that doesn't heal. It may affect up to 5 percent of patients with vulvar lichen sclerosus. In some cases lichen sclerosus is associated with differentiated vulval intraepithelial neoplasia (VIN).

Penile Lichen Sclerosus

In men, lichen sclerosus usually affects the tip of the penis, which becomes firm and white (also called balanitis xerotica perstans). The urethra may narrow such that it is difficult to pass urine, resulting in a thin stream. Sometimes the passage has to be widened with a special operation, called meatal dilation. Sexual function may be affected. The foreskin may be come difficult to retract (phimosis) and a circumcision may be needed.

Male genital lichen sclerosus is rare in men circumcised at birth. It has been suggested that it may be caused by chronic, intermittent damage by urine.

Penile lichen sclerosus may rarely predispose to penile intraepithelial neoplasia and penile cancer. Long-term follow-up is therefore recommended.

Other Skin Sites

Lichen sclerosus may also affect non-genital areas in 10 percent of patients with vulval disease. Six percent of men and women with lichen sclerosus on other sites have no genital involvement. One or more white patches may be found on the inner thigh, buttocks, under the breasts, neck, shoulders, and armpits. They often look like cigarette paper, with a wrinkled surface and waxy thickened feel. Less often they are scaly, bruised-looking, blistered, or ulcerated. In these sites, lichen sclerosus is generally not itchy and it does not appear to predispose to cancer.

What Is The Cause Of Lichen Sclerosus?

The cause of lichen sclerosus is not fully understood and may include genetic, hormonal, irritant, and infectious components. Lichen sclerosus is believed to relate to an autoimmune process, in which there are antibodies to a component of the skin. This is possibly extracellular matrix protein-1 (ECM-1) as antibodies to this protein have been detected in 75 percent to 80 percent of women with vulval lichen sclerosus.

Other autoimmune conditions such as thyroid disease (about 20 percent of patients), pernicious anemia, vitiligo, morphea, alopecia areata, and psoriasis are reported to be more frequent than expected in patients who have lichen sclerosus and in their families.

How Is It Diagnosed?

Often the diagnosis is made by a dermatologist or gynecologist after a careful clinical examination. A skin biopsy is frequently recommended to confirm the diagnosis, as there are characteristic histopathological findings in lichen sclerosus. One or more biopsies may be taken to rule out other possible explanations for the skin condition such as dermatitis, lichen planus and vulval intraepithelial neoplasia. Sometimes these disorders may co-exist with lichen sclerosus.

During follow-up, your specialist may decide to perform another biopsy to evaluate areas of concern.

Treatment

Strong topical steroid creams or ointments (especially clobetasol propionate) are very helpful for lichen sclerosus, especially when it affects genital areas. They should be applied very accurately as a thin smear to the affected areas for a few weeks or months. Overuse of steroid creams can result in skin thinning, red skin, and discomfort; this is uncommon when applied to mucosal surfaces alone. It is most important to follow instructions carefully and to attend follow-up appointments regularly.

Most patients will be told to apply the steroid cream once a day initially. The doctor should reassess the treated area after a few weeks as the response to treatment is quite variable. The itch often settles within a few days but it takes weeks to months for the appearance to return to normal. Once the lichen sclerosus has resolved or skin thinning due to the cream has arisen, the cream should be used less often. It may need to be continued on a regular basis (perhaps once a week) to prevent the lichen sclerosus recurring. In general, after initial more generous treatment, one 30-gram tube is expected to last about 6 to 12 months.

Wash gently in a shower or bath with plain water alone or with a non-soap cleanser. Try to avoid rubbing and scratching. Some patients find it helpful to apply an emollient cream or petrolatum several times a day to relieve dryness or itching.

If the first topical steroid is not well tolerated or ineffective, another one should be used. An ointment may be preferred to a cream (or vice versa).

Topical estrogen creams may be prescribed for atrophic vulvovaginitis (dry, thinned and sensitive vulval and vaginal tissues due to hormonal deficiency), to strengthen the tissues and to prevent fissuring.

There are a variety of other treatments occasionally prescribed as well or instead of steroid creams. These include calcipotriol cream, topical and systemic retinoids (acitretin), and systemic steroids.

The new immune modulating creams tacrolimus and pimecrolimus look promising for treating lichen sclerosus, but may be difficult to use because they tend to cause burning. There is also concern that these medications may have the potential to accelerate skin cancer formation in the presence of oncogenic human papilloma virus (genital warts).

Photodynamic therapy has also been reported to be of benefit, but the procedure may be very painful.

Experimentally, fat cells and platelet-rich plasma injected into affected areas have been reported to result in regeneration of normal skin.

If the vaginal opening has narrowed, it may need gentle stretching using dilators. Rarely, surgery is necessary to allow sexual intercourse. Unfortunately, the lichen sclerosus sometimes closes up the vaginal opening again after surgery has initially appeared successful.

Surgery

Surgical release of vulval and vaginal adhesions and scarring from vulval lichen sclerosus may occasionally be performed to reduce urination difficulties and allow intercourse. Procedures may include:

- Simple perineotomy (division of adhesions)

- Fenton procedure (an incision that is repaired transversely)

- Perineoplasty (excision of involved tissue and vaginal mucosal advancement)

Surgery to remove the entire vulva (vulvectomy) is reserved for the most severe cases or if there is vulvar cancer or pre-cancer (vulval intraepithelial neoplasia or VIN).

Chapter 31

Lupus

Defining Lupus

Lupus is one of many disorders of the immune system known as autoimmune diseases. In autoimmune diseases, the immune system turns against parts of the body it is designed to protect. This leads to inflammation and damage to various body tissues. Lupus can affect many parts of the body, including the joints, skin, kidneys, heart, lungs, blood vessels, and brain. Although people with the disease may have many different symptoms, some of the most common ones include extreme fatigue, painful or swollen joints (arthritis), unexplained fever, skin rashes, and kidney problems.

At present, there is no cure for lupus. However, lupus can be effectively treated with drugs, and most people with the disease can lead active, healthy lives. Lupus is characterized by periods of illness, called flares, and periods of wellness, or remission. Understanding how to prevent flares and how to treat them when they do occur helps people with lupus maintain better health. Intense research is underway, and scientists funded by the National Institutes of Health are continuing to make great strides in understanding the disease, which may ultimately lead to a cure.

Two of the major questions researchers are studying are who gets lupus and why. We know that many more women than men have lupus. Lupus is two to three times more common in

About This Chapter: Information in this chapter is from "Handout on Health: Systemic Lupus Erythematosus," National Institute of Arthritis and Musculoskeletal and Skin Diseases (www.niams.nih.gov), August 2011. Brand names included in this publication are provided as examples only, and their inclusion does not mean that these products are endorsed by the National Institutes of Health or any other government agency. Also, if a particular brand name is not mentioned, this does not mean or imply that the product is unsatisfactory.

African American women than in Caucasian women and is also more common in women of Hispanic, Asian, and Native-American descent. African-American and Hispanic women are also more likely to have active disease and serious organ system involvement. In addition, lupus can run in families, but the risk that a child or a brother or sister of a patient will also have lupus is still quite low. It is difficult to estimate how many people in the United States have the disease, because its symptoms vary widely and its onset is often hard to pinpoint.

There are several kinds of lupus:

Systemic Lupus Erythematosus: Systemic lupus erythematosus (SLE) is the form of the disease that most people are referring to when they say "lupus." The word "systemic" means the disease can affect many parts of the body. The symptoms of SLE may be mild or serious. Although SLE usually first affects people between the ages of 15 and 45 years, it can occur in childhood or later in life as well. This chapter focuses on SLE.

Discoid Lupus Erythematosus: This is a chronic skin disorder in which a red, raised rash appears on the face, scalp, or elsewhere. The raised areas may become thick and scaly and may cause scarring. The rash may last for days or years and may recur. A small percentage of people with discoid lupus have or develop SLE later.

Subacute Cutaneous Lupus Erythematosus: This type of lupus refers to skin lesions that appear on parts of the body exposed to sun. The lesions do not cause scarring.

Drug-Induced Lupus: This form of lupus caused by medications. Many different drugs can cause drug-induced lupus. Symptoms are similar to those of SLE (arthritis, rash, fever, and chest pain), and they typically go away completely when the drug is stopped. The kidneys and brain are rarely involved.

Neonatal Lupus: This type of lupus is a rare disease that can occur in newborn babies of women with SLE, Sjögren's syndrome, or no disease at all. Scientists suspect that neonatal lupus is caused in part by autoantibodies in the mother's blood called anti-Ro (SSA) and anti-La (SSB). Autoantibodies ("auto" means self) are blood proteins that act against the body's own parts. At birth, the babies have a skin rash, liver problems, and low blood counts. These symptoms gradually go away over several months. In rare instances, babies with neonatal lupus may have congenital heart block, a serious heart problem in which the formation of fibrous tissue in the baby's heart interferes with the electrical impulses that affect heart rhythm. Neonatal lupus is rare, and most infants of mothers with SLE are entirely healthy. All women who are pregnant and known to have anti-Ro (SSA) or anti-La (SSB) antibodies should be monitored by echocardiograms (a test that monitors the heart and surrounding blood vessels) during the 16th and 30th weeks of pregnancy.

It is important for women with SLE or other related autoimmune disorders to be under a doctor's care during pregnancy. Doctors can now identify mothers at highest risk for complications, allowing for prompt treatment of the infant at or before birth. SLE can also flare during pregnancy, and prompt treatment can keep the mother healthier longer.

Understanding What Causes Lupus

Lupus is a complex disease, and its cause is unknown.

In studies of identical twins—who are born with the exact same genes—when one twin has lupus, the other twin has a 24-percent chance of developing it. This and other research suggests that genetics plays an important role, but it also shows that genes alone do not determine who gets lupus, and that other factors play a role. Some of the factors scientists are studying include sunlight, stress, hormones, cigarette smoke, certain drugs, and infectious agents such as viruses. Recent research has confirmed that one virus, Epstein-Barr virus (EBV), which causes mononucleosis, is a cause of lupus in genetically susceptible people.

Scientists believe there is no single gene that predisposes people to lupus. Rather, studies suggest that a number of different genes may be involved in determining a person's likelihood of developing the disease, which tissues and organs are affected, and the severity of disease.

In lupus, the body's immune system does not work as it should. A healthy immune system produces proteins called antibodies and specific cells called lymphocytes that help fight and destroy viruses, bacteria, and other foreign substances that invade the body. In lupus, the immune system produces antibodies against the body's healthy cells and tissues. These antibodies, called autoantibodies, contribute to the inflammation of various parts of the body and can cause damage to organs and tissues. The most common type of autoantibody that develops in people with lupus is called an antinuclear antibody (ANA) because it reacts with parts of the cell's nucleus (command center). Doctors and scientists do not yet understand all of the factors that cause inflammation and tissue damage in lupus, and researchers are actively exploring them.

Symptoms Of Lupus

Each person with lupus has slightly different symptoms that can range from mild to severe and may come and go over time. However, some of the most common symptoms of lupus include painful or swollen joints (arthritis), unexplained fever, and extreme fatigue. A characteristic red skin rash—the so-called butterfly or malar rash—may appear across the nose and cheeks. Rashes may also occur on the face and ears, upper arms, shoulders, chest, and hands. Because many people with lupus are sensitive to sunlight (called photosensitivity), skin rashes often first develop or worsen after sun exposure.

What's It Mean?

Anemia: A decrease in red blood cells.

Arthritis: Painful or swollen joints.

Autoantibodies: Proteins in the blood that turn against healthy body parts.

Edema: Swelling—can occur around the eyes or in the legs with lupus.

Epstein-Barr Virus: A cause of lupus in some people.

Malar Rash: Also called butterfly rash, a red skin rash across the nose and cheeks.

Nephritis: Inflammation of the kidneys.

Photosensitivity: Sensitivity to sunlight.

Pleuritis: Inflammation of the chest cavity lining that can cause pain with breathing and come with pneumonia.

Rheumatologist: A doctor who specializes in rheumatic diseases (arthritis and other inflammatory disorders, often involving the immune system).

Common Symptoms Of Lupus

The following are some common symptoms of lupus:

- Painful or swollen joints and muscle pain

- Unexplained fever

- Red rashes, most commonly on the face

- Chest pain upon deep breathing

- Unusual loss of hair

- Pale or purple fingers or toes from cold or stress (Raynaud's phenomenon)

- Sensitivity to the sun

- Swelling (edema) in legs or around eyes

- Mouth ulcers

- Swollen glands

- Extreme fatigue

Other symptoms of lupus include chest pain, hair loss, anemia (a decrease in red blood cells), mouth ulcers, and pale or purple fingers and toes from cold and stress. Some people also experience headaches, dizziness, depression, confusion, or seizures. New symptoms may continue to appear years after the initial diagnosis, and different symptoms can occur at different times. In some people with lupus, only one system of the body, such as the skin or joints, is affected. Other people experience symptoms in many parts of their body. Just how seriously a body system is affected varies from person to person. The following systems in the body also can be affected by lupus:

- **Kidneys:** Inflammation of the kidneys (nephritis) can impair their ability to get rid of waste products and other toxins from the body effectively. There is usually no pain associated with kidney involvement, although some patients may notice dark urine and swelling around their eyes, legs, ankles, or fingers. Most often, the only indication of kidney disease is an abnormal urine or blood test. Because the kidneys are so important to overall health, lupus affecting the kidneys generally requires intensive drug treatment to prevent permanent damage.

- **Lungs:** Some people with lupus develop pleuritis, an inflammation of the lining of the chest cavity that causes chest pain, particularly with breathing. Patients with lupus also may get pneumonia.

- **Central Nervous System:** In some patients, lupus affects the brain or central nervous system. This can cause headaches, dizziness, depression, memory disturbances, vision problems, seizures, stroke, or changes in behavior.

- **Blood Vessels:** Blood vessels may become inflamed (vasculitis), affecting the way blood circulates through the body. The inflammation may be mild and may not require treatment or may be severe and require immediate attention.

- **Blood:** People with lupus may develop anemia, leukopenia (a decreased number of white blood cells), or thrombocytopenia (a decrease in the number of platelets in the blood, which assist in clotting). People with lupus who have a type of autoantibody called antiphospholipid antibodies have an increased risk of blood clots.

- **Heart:** In some people with lupus, inflammation can occur in the heart itself (myocarditis and endocarditis) or the membrane that surrounds it (pericarditis), causing chest pains or other symptoms. Endocarditis can damage the heart valves, causing the valve surface to thicken and develop growths, which can cause heart murmurs. However, this usually doesn't affect the valves' function.

Diagnosing Lupus

Diagnosing lupus can be difficult. It may take months or even years for doctors to piece together the symptoms to diagnose this complex disease accurately. Making a correct diagnosis of lupus requires knowledge and awareness on the part of the doctor and good communication on the part of the patient. Giving the doctor a complete, accurate medical history (for example, what health problems you have had and for how long) is critical to the process of diagnosis. This information, along with a physical examination and the results of laboratory tests, helps the doctor consider other diseases that may mimic lupus, or determine if you truly have the disease. Reaching a diagnosis may take time as new symptoms appear.

No single test can determine whether a person has lupus, but several laboratory tests may help the doctor to confirm a diagnosis of lupus or rule out other causes for a person's symptoms. The most useful tests identify certain autoantibodies often present in the blood of people with lupus. For example, the antinuclear antibody (ANA) test is commonly used to look for autoantibodies that react against components of the nucleus, or "command center," of the body's cells.

Other laboratory tests are used to monitor the progress of the disease once it has been diagnosed. A complete blood count, urinalysis, blood chemistries, and the erythrocyte sedimentation rate (ESR) test (a test to measure inflammation) can provide valuable information. Another common test measures the blood level of a group of substances called complement, which help antibodies fight invaders. A low level of complement could mean the substance is being used up because of an immune response in the body, such as that which occurs during a flare of lupus. X-rays and other imaging tests can help doctors see the organs affected by SLE.

Diagnostic Tools For Lupus

- Medical history
- Complete physical examination
- Laboratory tests:
    1. Complete blood count (CBC)
    2. Erythrocyte sedimentation rate (ESR)
    3. Urinalysis
    4. Blood chemistries
    5. Complement levels
    6. Antinuclear antibody test (ANA)

7. Other autoantibody tests (anti-DNA, anti-Sm, anti-RNP, anti-Ro [SSA], anti-La [SSB])

8. Anticardiolipin antibody test

- Skin biopsy

- Kidney biopsy

Treating Lupus

Diagnosing and treating lupus often require a team effort between the patient and several types of health care professionals. A person with lupus can go to his or her family doctor or internist, or can visit a rheumatologist. A rheumatologist is a doctor who specializes in rheumatic diseases (arthritis and other inflammatory disorders, often involving the immune system). Clinical immunologists (doctors specializing in immune system disorders) may also treat people with lupus. As treatment progresses, other professionals often help. These may include nurses, psychologists, social workers, nephrologists (doctors who treat kidney disease), cardiologists (doctors specializing in the heart and blood vessels), hematologists (doctors specializing in blood disorders), endocrinologists (doctors specializing in problems related to the glands and hormones), dermatologists (doctors who treat skin disease), and neurologists (doctors specializing in disorders of the nervous system).

Once lupus has been diagnosed, the doctor will develop a treatment plan based on the patient's age, sex, health, symptoms, and lifestyle. Treatment plans are tailored to the individual's needs and may change over time. In developing a treatment plan, the doctor has several goals: to prevent flares, to treat them when they do occur, and to minimize organ damage and complications. The doctor and patient should reevaluate the plan regularly to ensure it is as effective as possible.

NSAIDs: For people with joint or chest pain or fever, drugs that decrease inflammation, called nonsteroidal anti-inflammatory drugs (NSAIDs), are often used. Although some NSAIDs, such as ibuprofen and naproxen, are available over the counter, a doctor's prescription is necessary for others. NSAIDs may be used alone or in combination with other types of drugs to control pain, swelling, and fever. Even though some NSAIDs may be purchased without a prescription, it is important that they be taken under a doctor's direction.

Antimalarials: Antimalarials are another type of drug commonly used to treat lupus. These drugs were originally used to treat malaria, but doctors have found that they also are useful for lupus. A common antimalarial used to treat lupus is hydroxychloroquine (Plaquenil). It may be used alone or in combination with other drugs and generally is used to treat fatigue, joint pain, skin rashes, and inflammation of the lungs.

Corticosteroids: The mainstay of lupus treatment involves the use of corticosteroid hormones, such as prednisone (Deltasone), hydrocortisone, methylprednisolone (Medrol), and dexamethasone (Decadron, Hexadrol). Corticosteroids are related to cortisol, which is a natural anti-inflammatory hormone. They work by rapidly suppressing inflammation. Corticosteroids can be given by mouth, in creams applied to the skin, by injection, or by intravenous (IV) infusion (dripping the drug into the vein through a small tube). Because they are potent drugs, the doctor will seek the lowest dose with the greatest benefit. Short-term side effects of corticosteroids include swelling, increased appetite, and weight gain. These side effects generally stop when the drug is stopped. It is dangerous to stop taking corticosteroids suddenly, so it is very important that the doctor and patient work together in changing the corticosteroid dose. Sometimes doctors give very large amounts of corticosteroid by vein over a brief period of time (days) ("bolus" or "pulse" therapy). With this treatment, the typical side effects are less likely and slow withdrawal is unnecessary.

Immunosuppressives: For some patients whose kidneys or central nervous systems are affected by lupus, a type of drug called an immunosuppressive may be used. Immunosuppressives, such as cyclophosphamide (Cytoxan) and mycophenolate mofetil (CellCept), restrain the overactive immune system by blocking the production of immune cells. These drugs may be given by mouth or by IV infusion. Side effects may include nausea, vomiting, hair loss, bladder problems, decreased fertility, and increased risk of cancer and infection. The risk for side effects increases with the length of treatment. As with other treatments for lupus, there is a risk of relapse after the immunosuppressives have been stopped.

BLyS-Specific Inhibitors: Belimumab (Benlysta), a B-lymphocyte stimulator (BLyS) protein inhibitor, was approved by the U.S. Food and Drug Administration (FDA) in March 2011 for patients with lupus who are receiving other standard therapies, including those listed above. Given by IV infusion, it may reduce the number of abnormal B cells thought to be a problem in lupus.

In studies conducted so far, African American patients and patients of African heritage did not appear to respond to belimumab. An additional study of this patient population will be conducted to further evaluate belimumab in this subgroup of lupus patients. However, this difference in response to a treatment may be another indicator of the various ways that the disease affects different patients.

Other Therapies: In some patients, methotrexate (Folex, Mexate, Rheumatrex), a disease-modifying antirheumatic drug, may be used to help control the disease. Other treatments may include hormonal therapies such as dehydroepiandrosterone (DHEA) and intravenous immunoglobulin (proteins derived from human blood), which may be useful for controlling lupus when other treatments haven't worked.

Alternative And Complementary Therapies: Because of the nature and cost of the medications used to treat lupus and the potential for serious side effects, many patients seek other ways of treating the disease. Some alternative approaches people have tried include special diets, nutritional supplements, fish oils, ointments and creams, chiropractic treatment, and homeopathy. Although these methods may not be harmful in and of themselves and may be associated with symptomatic or psychosocial benefit, no research to date shows that they affect the disease process or prevent organ damage. Some alternative or complementary approaches may help the patient cope or reduce some of the stress associated with living with a chronic illness. If the doctor feels the approach has value and will not be harmful, it can be incorporated into the patient's treatment plan. However, it is important not to neglect regular health care or treatment of serious symptoms. An open dialogue between the patient and doctor about the relative values of complementary and alternative therapies allows the patient to make an informed choice about treatment options.

Lupus And Quality Of Life

Despite the symptoms of lupus and the potential side effects of treatment, people with lupus can maintain a high quality of life overall. One key to managing lupus is to understand the disease and its impact. Learning to recognize the warning signs of a flare can help the patient take steps to ward it off or reduce its intensity. Many people with lupus experience increased fatigue, pain, a rash, fever, abdominal discomfort, headache, or dizziness just before a flare. Developing strategies to prevent flares can also be helpful, such as learning to recognize your warning signals and maintaining good communication with your doctor.

It is also important for people with lupus to receive regular health care, instead of seeking help only when symptoms worsen. Results from a medical exam and laboratory work on a regular basis allow the doctor to note any changes and to identify and treat flares early. The treatment plan, which is tailored to the individual's specific needs and circumstances, can be adjusted accordingly. If new symptoms are identified early, treatments may be more effective. Other concerns also can be addressed at regular checkups. The doctor can provide guidance about such issues as the use of sunscreens, stress reduction, and the importance of structured exercise and rest, as well as birth control and family planning. Because people with lupus can be more susceptible to infections, the doctor may recommend yearly influenza vaccinations or pneumococcal vaccinations for some patients.

Women with lupus should receive regular preventive health care, such as gynecological and breast examinations. Men with lupus should have the prostate-specific antigen (PSA) test. Both men and women need to have their blood pressure and cholesterol checked on a regular basis. If a person is taking corticosteroids or antimalarial medications, an eye exam should be done at least yearly to screen for and treat eye problems.

Staying healthy requires extra effort and care for people with lupus, so it becomes especially important to develop strategies for maintaining wellness. Wellness involves close attention to the body, mind, and spirit. One of the primary goals of wellness for people with lupus is coping with the stress of having a chronic disorder. Effective stress management varies from person to person. Some approaches that may help include exercise, relaxation techniques such as meditation, and setting priorities for spending time and energy.

Developing and maintaining a good support system is also important. A support system may include family, friends, medical professionals, community organizations, and support groups. Participating in a support group can provide emotional help, boost self-esteem and morale, and help develop or improve coping skills.

Warning Signs Of A Flare

The warning signs of a lupus flare include the following:

- Increased fatigue
- Pain
- Rash
- Fever
- Abdominal discomfort
- Headache
- Dizziness

Preventing A Flare

- Learn to recognize your warning signals.
- Maintain good communication with your doctor.

Learning more about lupus may also help. Studies have shown that patients who are well-informed and participate actively in their own care experience less pain, make fewer visits to the doctor, build self-confidence, and remain more active.

Tips For Working With Your Doctor

- Seek a health care provider who is familiar with SLE and who will listen to and address your concerns.
- Provide complete, accurate medical information.
- Make a list of your questions and concerns in advance.
- Be honest and share your point of view with the health care provider.
- Ask for clarification or further explanation if you need it.
- Talk to other members of the health care team, such as nurses, therapists, or pharmacists.
- Do not hesitate to discuss sensitive subjects (for example, birth control, intimacy) with your doctor.
- Discuss any treatment changes with your doctor before making them.

Pregnancy For Women With Lupus

Although pregnancy in women with lupus is considered high risk, most women with lupus carry their babies safely to the end of their pregnancy. Women with lupus in general have a higher rate of miscarriage and premature births compared with the general population. In addition, women who have antiphospholipid antibodies are at a greater risk of miscarriage in the second trimester because of their increased risk of blood clotting in the placenta. Lupus patients with a history of kidney disease have a higher risk of preeclampsia (hypertension with a buildup of excess watery fluid in cells or tissues of the body). Pregnancy counseling and planning before pregnancy are important. Ideally, a woman should have no signs or symptoms of lupus and be taking no medications for at least six months before she becomes pregnant.

Some women may experience a mild to moderate flare during or after their pregnancy; others do not. Pregnant women with lupus, especially those taking corticosteroids, also are more likely to develop high blood pressure, diabetes, hyperglycemia (high blood sugar), and kidney complications, so regular care and good nutrition during pregnancy are essential. It is also advisable to have access to a neonatal (newborn) intensive care unit at the time of delivery in case the baby requires special medical attention.

Chapter 32

Melanoma And
Other Skin Cancers

Skin cancer is the most common type of cancer in the United States. Each year, more than 68,000 Americans are diagnosed with melanoma, and another 48,000 are diagnosed with an early form of the disease that involves only the top layer of skin. Also, more than 2 million people are treated for basal cell or squamous cell skin cancer each year. Basal cell skin cancer is several times more common than squamous cell skin cancer.

Learning about medical care for skin cancer can help you take an active part in making choices about your care. This chapter tells about the following:

- Diagnosis and staging

- Treatment

- Follow-up care

- How to prevent another skin cancer from forming

- How to do a skin self-exam

This chapter has lists of questions that you may want to ask your doctor. Many people find it helpful to take a list of questions to a doctor visit. To help remember what your doctor says, you can take notes.

You may also want to have a family member or friend go with you when you talk with the doctor—to take notes, ask questions, or just listen.

About This Chapter: Information in this chapter is from "What You Need To Know About Melanoma And Other Skin Cancers," National Cancer Institute (www.cancer.gov), January 11, 2011.

The Skin

Your skin protects your body from heat, injury, and infection. It also protects your body from damage caused by ultraviolet (UV) radiation (such as from the sun or sunlamps).

Your skin stores water and fat. It helps control body heat. Also, your skin makes vitamin D. Skin contains two main layers:

- **Epidermis:** The epidermis is the top layer of your skin. It's mostly made of flat cells called *squamous cells*. Below the squamous cells deeper in the epidermis are round cells called *basal cells*. Cells called *melanocytes* are scattered among the basal cells. They are in the deepest part of the epidermis. Melanocytes make the pigment (color) found in skin. When skin is exposed to UV radiation, melanocytes make more pigment, causing the skin to darken, or tan.

- **Dermis:** The dermis is the layer under the epidermis. The dermis contains many types of cells and structures, such as blood vessels, lymph vessels, and glands. Some of these glands make sweat, which helps cool your body. Other glands make sebum. Sebum is an oily substance that helps keep your skin from drying out. Sweat and sebum reach the surface of your skin through tiny openings called pores.

Cancer Cells

Cancer begins in cells, the building blocks that make up tissues. Tissues make up the skin and other organs of the body.

Normal cells grow and divide to form new cells as the body needs them. When normal cells grow old or get damaged, they usually die, and new cells take their place.

But sometimes this process goes wrong. New cells form when the body doesn't need them, and old or damaged cells don't die as they should. The buildup of extra cells often forms a mass of tissue called a growth or tumor.

Growths on the skin can be benign (not cancer) or malignant (cancer). Benign growths are not as harmful as malignant growths.

- **Benign Growths** (such as moles):
  - Are rarely a threat to life
  - Generally can be removed and usually don't grow back
  - Don't invade the tissues around them
  - Don't spread to other parts of the body

- **Malignant Growths** (such as melanoma, basal cell cancer, or squamous cell cancer):

  - May be a threat to life

  - Often can be removed but sometimes grow back

  - May invade and damage nearby organs and tissues

  - May spread to other parts of the body

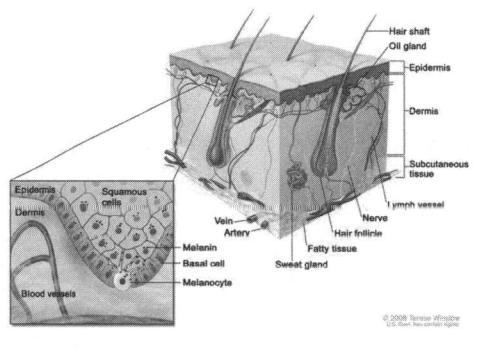

Figure 32.1. Melanoma anatomy. (Source: © 2008 Terese Winslow, U.S. Govt. has certain rights.)

Types of Skin Cancer

Skin cancers are named for the type of cells that become malignant (cancer). The following are the three most common types:

- **Melanoma:** Melanoma begins in melanocytes (pigment cells). Most melanocytes are in the skin. Melanoma can occur on any skin surface. In men, it's often found on the skin on the head, on the neck, or between the shoulders and the hips. In women, it's often found on the skin on the lower legs or between the shoulders and the hips. Melanoma is rare in people with dark skin. When it does develop in people with dark skin, it's usually found under the fingernails, under the toenails, on the palms of the hands, or on the soles of the feet.

- **Basal Cell Skin Cancer:** Basal cell skin cancer begins in the basal cell layer of the skin. It usually occurs in places that have been in the sun. For example, the face is the most common place to find basal cell skin cancer. In people with fair skin, basal cell skin cancer is the most common type of skin cancer.

- **Squamous Cell Skin Cancer:** Squamous cell skin cancer begins in squamous cells. In people with dark skin, squamous cell skin cancer is the most common type of skin cancer, and it's usually found in places that are not in the sun, such as the legs or feet. However, in people with fair skin, squamous cell skin cancer usually occurs on parts of the skin that have been in the sun, such as the head, face, ears, and neck.

Unlike moles, skin cancer can invade the normal tissue nearby. Also, skin cancer can spread throughout the body. Melanoma is more likely than other skin cancers to spread to other parts of the body. Squamous cell skin cancer sometimes spreads to other parts of the body, but basal cell skin cancer rarely does.

When skin cancer cells do spread, they break away from the original growth and enter blood vessels or lymph vessels. The cancer cells may be found in nearby lymph nodes. The cancer cells can also spread to other tissues and attach there to form new tumors that may damage those tissues.

The spread of cancer is called metastasis. See the "Staging" section for information about skin cancer that has spread.

Risk Factors

When you're told that you have skin cancer, it's natural to wonder what may have caused the disease. The main risk factor for skin cancer is exposure to sunlight (UV radiation), but there are also other risk factors. A risk factor is something that may increase the chance of getting a disease.

People with certain risk factors are more likely than others to develop skin cancer. Some risk factors vary for the different types of skin cancer.

What's It Mean?

Basal Cells: Skin cells located deep in the epidermis.

Benign: Not cancerous.

Skin Biopsy: Small sample sent to a lab to help diagnose disease.

Malignant: Cancerous.

Melanocytes: Cells that give skin its color (pigment).

Squamous Cells: Skin cells located in the surface of the epidermis.

Source: NCI, January 11, 2011.

Risks For Any Type Of Skin Cancer

Studies have shown that the following are risk factors for the three most common types of skin cancer:

- **Sunlight:** Sunlight is a source of UV radiation. It's the most important risk factor for any type of skin cancer. The sun's rays cause skin damage that can lead to cancer.

- **Severe, Blistering Sunburns:** People who have had at least one severe, blistering sunburn are at increased risk of skin cancer. Although people who burn easily are more likely to have had sunburns as a child, sunburns during adulthood also increase the risk of skin cancer.

- **Lifetime Sun Exposure:** The total amount of sun exposure over a lifetime is a risk factor for skin cancer.

- **Tanning:** Although a tan slightly lowers the risk of sunburn, even people who tan well without sunburning have a higher risk of skin cancer because of more lifetime sun exposure.

Sunlight can be reflected by sand, water, snow, ice, and pavement. The sun's rays can get through clouds, windshields, windows, and light clothing.

In the United States, skin cancer is more common where the sun is strong. For example, more people in Texas than Minnesota get skin cancer. Also, the sun is stronger at higher elevations, such as in the mountains.

Doctors encourage people to limit their exposure to sunlight.

- **Sunlamps And Tanning Booths:** Artificial sources of UV radiation, such as sunlamps and tanning booths, can cause skin damage and skin cancer. Health care providers strongly encourage people, especially young people, to avoid using sunlamps and tanning booths. The risk of skin cancer is greatly increased by using sunlamps and tanning booths before age 30.

- **Personal History:** People who have had melanoma have an increased risk of developing other melanomas. Also, people who have had basal cell or squamous cell skin cancer have an increased risk of developing another skin cancer of any type.

- **Family History:** Melanoma sometimes runs in families. Having two or more close relatives (mother, father, sister, brother, or child) who have had this disease is a risk factor for developing melanoma. Other types of skin cancer also sometimes run in families. Rarely, members of a family will have an inherited disorder, such as *xeroderma pigmentosum* or nevoid basal cell carcinoma syndrome, that makes the skin more sensitive to the sun and increases the risk of skin cancer.

- **Skin That Burns Easily:** Having fair (pale) skin that burns in the sun easily, blue or gray eyes, red or blond hair, or many freckles increases the risk of skin cancer.

- **Certain Medical Conditions Or Medicines:** Medical conditions or medicines (such as some antibiotics, hormones, or antidepressants) that make your skin more sensitive to the sun increase the risk of skin cancer. Also, medical conditions or medicines that suppress the immune system increase the risk of skin cancer.

Other Risk Factors For Melanoma

The following risk factors increase the risk of melanoma:

- **Dysplastic Nevus:** A dysplastic nevus is a type of mole that looks different from a common mole. A dysplastic nevus may be bigger than a common mole, and its color, surface, and border may be different. It's usually wider than a pea and may be longer than a peanut. A dysplastic nevus can have a mixture of several colors, from pink to dark brown. Usually, it's flat with a smooth, slightly scaly or pebbly surface, and it has an irregular edge that may fade into the surrounding skin. A dysplastic nevus is more likely than a common mole to turn into cancer. However, most do not change into melanoma. A doctor will remove a dysplastic nevus if it looks like it might have changed into melanoma.

- **More Than 50 Common Moles:** Usually, a common mole is smaller than a pea, has an even color (pink, tan, or brown), and is round or oval with a smooth surface. Having many common moles increases the risk of developing melanoma.

Other Risk Factors For Both Basal Cell And Squamous Cell Skin Cancers

The following risk factors increase the risk of basal cell and squamous cell skin cancers:

- **Old scars, burns, ulcers, or areas of inflammation** on the skin

- **Exposure to arsenic** at work

- **Radiation therapy**

Other Risk Factors For Squamous Cell Cancer

The risk of squamous cell skin cancer is increased by the following:

- **Actinic Keratosis:** Actinic keratosis is a type of flat, scaly growth on the skin. It is most often found on areas exposed to the sun, especially the face and the backs of the hands.

The growth may appear as a rough red or brown patch on the skin. It may also appear as cracking or peeling of the lower lip that does not heal. Without treatment, this scaly growth may turn into squamous cell skin cancer.

- **HPV (Human Papillomavirus):** Certain types of HPV can infect the skin and may increase the risk of squamous cell skin cancer. These HPVs are different from the HPV types that cause cervical cancer and other cancers in the female and male genital areas.

Symptoms Of Melanoma

Often the first sign of melanoma is a change in the shape, color, size, or feel of an existing mole. Melanoma may also appear as a new mole. Thinking of "ABCDE" can help you remember what to look for:

- **Asymmetry:** The shape of one half does not match the other half.

- **Border That Is Irregular:** The edges are often ragged, notched, or blurred in outline. The pigment may spread into the surrounding skin.

- **Color That Is Uneven:** Shades of black, brown, and tan may be present. Areas of white, gray, red, pink, or blue may also be seen.

- **Diameter:** There is a change in size, usually an increase. Melanomas can be tiny, but most are larger than the size of a pea (larger than 6 millimeters or about 1/4 inch).

- **Evolving:** The mole has changed over the past few weeks or months.

Melanomas can vary greatly in how they look. Many show all of the ABCDE features. However, some may show changes or abnormal areas in only one or two of the ABCDE features.

In more advanced melanoma, the texture of the mole may change. The skin on the surface may break down and look scraped. It may become hard or lumpy. The surface may ooze or bleed. Sometimes the melanoma is itchy, tender, or painful.

Symptoms Of Basal Cell And Squamous Cell Skin Cancers

A change on the skin is the most common sign of skin cancer. This may be a new growth, a sore that doesn't heal, or a change in an old growth. Not all skin cancers look the same. Usually, skin cancer is not painful. Common symptoms of basal cell or squamous cell skin cancer include these:

- A lump that is small, smooth, shiny, pale, or waxy
- A lump that is firm and red
- A sore or lump that bleeds or develops a crust or a scab
- A flat red spot that is rough, dry, or scaly and may become itchy or tender
- A red or brown patch that is rough and scaly

Diagnosis

If you have a change on your skin, your doctor must find out whether or not the problem is from cancer. You may need to see a dermatologist, a doctor who has special training in the diagnosis and treatment of skin problems.

Your doctor will check the skin all over your body to see if other unusual growths are present.

If your doctor suspects that a spot on the skin is cancer, you may need a biopsy. For a biopsy, your doctor may remove all or part of the skin that does not look normal. The sample goes to a lab. A pathologist checks the sample under a microscope. Sometimes it's helpful for more than one pathologist to check the tissue for cancer cells.

You may have the biopsy in a doctor's office or as an outpatient in a clinic or hospital. You'll probably have local anesthesia. There are four common types of skin biopsies:

- **Shave Biopsy:** The doctor uses a thin, sharp blade to shave off the abnormal growth.
- **Punch Biopsy:** The doctor uses a sharp, hollow tool to remove a circle of tissue from the abnormal area.
- **Incisional Biopsy:** The doctor uses a scalpel to remove part of the growth.
- **Excisional Biopsy:** The doctor uses a scalpel to remove the entire growth and some tissue around it. This type of biopsy is most commonly used for growths that appear to be melanoma.

Staging

If the biopsy shows that you have skin cancer, your doctor needs to learn the stage (extent) of the disease to help you choose the best treatment. The stage is based on these factors:

- The size (width) of the growth
- How deeply it has grown beneath the top layer of skin
- Whether cancer cells have spread to nearby lymph nodes or to other parts of the body

You may want to ask your doctor these questions before having a biopsy:

- Which type of biopsy do you suggest for me?
- How will the biopsy be done?
- Will I have to go to the hospital?
- How long will it take? Will I be awake? Will it hurt?
- Will the entire growth be removed?
- Are there any risks? What are the chances of infection or bleeding after the biopsy?
- Will there be a scar? If so, what will it look like?
- How soon will I know the results?
- If I do have cancer, who will talk with me about treatment?

Source: NCI, January 11, 2011

When skin cancer spreads from its original place to another part of the body, the new tumor has the same kind of abnormal cells and the same name as the primary (original) tumor. For example, if skin cancer spreads to the lung, the cancer cells in the lung are actually skin cancer cells. The disease is metastatic skin cancer, not lung cancer. For that reason, it's treated as skin cancer, not as lung cancer. Doctors sometimes call the new tumor "distant" disease.

Blood tests and an imaging test such as a chest X-ray, a CT scan, an MRI, or a PET scan may be used to check for the spread of skin cancer. For example, if a melanoma growth is thick, your doctor may order blood tests and an imaging test.

For squamous cell skin cancer or melanoma, the doctor will also check the lymph nodes near the cancer on the skin. If one or more lymph nodes near the skin cancer are enlarged (or if the lymph node looks enlarged on an imaging test), your doctor may use a thin needle to remove a sample of cells from the lymph node (fine-needle aspiration biopsy). A pathologist will check the sample for cancer cells.

Even if the nearby lymph nodes are not enlarged, the nodes may contain cancer cells. The stage is sometimes not known until after surgery to remove the growth and one or more nearby lymph nodes. For thick melanoma, surgeons may use a method called sentinel lymph node biopsy to remove the lymph node most likely to have cancer cells. Cancer cells may appear first in the sentinel node before spreading to other lymph nodes and other places in the body.

Stages Of Melanoma

The following are the stages of melanoma:

- **Stage 0:** The melanoma involves only the top layer of skin. It is called melanoma in situ.

- **Stage I:** The tumor is no more than 1 millimeter thick (about the width of the tip of a sharpened pencil.) The surface may appear broken down. Or, the tumor is between 1 and 2 millimeters thick, and the surface is not broken down.

- **Stage II:** The tumor is between 1 and 2 millimeters thick, and the surface appears broken down. Or, the thickness of the tumor is more than 2 millimeters, and the surface may appear broken down.

- **Stage III:** The melanoma cells have spread to at least one nearby lymph node. Or, the melanoma cells have spread from the original tumor to tissues nearby.

- **Stage IV:** Cancer cells have spread to the lung or other organs, skin areas, or lymph nodes far away from the original growth. Melanoma commonly spreads to other parts of the skin, tissue under the skin, lymph nodes, and lungs. It can also spread to the liver, brain, bones, and other organs.

Stages Of Other Skin Cancers

The following are the stages of basal cell and squamous cell skin cancers:

- **Stage 0:** The cancer involves only the top layer of skin. It is called carcinoma in situ.

  Bowen disease is an early form of squamous cell skin cancer. It usually looks like a reddish, scaly or thickened patch on the skin. If not treated, the cancer may grow deeper into the skin.

- **Stage I:** The growth is as large as 2 centimeters wide (more than three-quarters of an inch or about the size of a peanut).

- **Stage II:** The growth is larger than 2 centimeters wide.

- **Stage III:** The cancer has invaded below the skin to cartilage, muscle, or bone. Or, cancer cells have spread to nearby lymph nodes. Cancer cells have not spread to other places in the body.

- **Stage IV:** The cancer has spread to other places in the body. Basal cell cancer rarely spreads to other parts of the body, but squamous cell cancer sometimes spreads to lymph nodes and other organs.

Merkel Cell Carcinoma

Merkel cell carcinoma is a very rare disease in which malignant (cancer) cells form in the skin.

Merkel cells are found in the top layer of the skin. These cells are very close to the nerve endings that receive the sensation of touch. Merkel cell carcinoma, also called neuroendocrine carcinoma of the skin or trabecular cancer, is a very rare type of skin cancer that forms when Merkel cells grow out of control. Merkel cell carcinoma starts most often in areas of skin exposed to the sun, especially the head and neck, as well as the arms, legs, and trunk.

Merkel cell carcinoma tends to grow quickly and to metastasize (spread) at an early stage. It usually spreads first to nearby lymph nodes and then may spread to lymph nodes or skin in distant parts of the body, lungs, brain, bones, or other organs.

Sun exposure and having a weak immune system can affect the risk of developing Merkel cell carcinoma.

Anything that increases your risk of getting a disease is called a risk factor. Having a risk factor does not mean that you will get cancer; not having risk factors doesn't mean that you will not get cancer. People who think they may be at risk should discuss this with their doctor. Risk factors for Merkel cell carcinoma include the following:

- Being exposed to a lot of natural sunlight
- Being exposed to artificial sunlight, such as from tanning beds or psoralen and ultraviolet A (PUVA) therapy for psoriasis
- Having an immune system weakened by disease, such as chronic lymphocytic leukemia or HIV infection
- Taking drugs that make the immune system less active, such as after an organ transplant
- Having a history of other types of cancer
- Being older than 50 years, male, or white

Merkel cell carcinoma usually appears as a single painless lump on sun-exposed skin.

This and other changes in the skin may be caused by Merkel cell carcinoma. Other conditions may cause the same symptoms. A doctor should be consulted if changes in the skin are seen.

Merkel cell carcinoma usually appears on sun-exposed skin as a single lump that has these characteristics:

- Fast-growing
- Painless
- Firm and dome-shaped or raised
- Red or violet in color

Source: PDQ® Cancer Information Summary. National Cancer Institute; Bethesda, MD. Merkel Cell Carcinoma Treatment (PDQ): Patient Version. Updated 03/2012. Available at: http://cancer.gov. Accessed February 9, 2013.

Treatment

Treatment for skin cancer depends on the type and stage of the disease, the size and place of the tumor, and your general health and medical history. In most cases, the goal of treatment is to remove or destroy the cancer completely. Most skin cancers can be cured if found and treated early.

Sometimes all of the skin cancer is removed during the biopsy. In such cases, no more treatment is needed.

If you do need more treatment, your doctor can describe your treatment choices and what to expect. You and your doctor can work together to develop a treatment plan that meets your needs.

Surgery is the usual treatment for people with skin cancer. In some cases, the doctor may suggest chemotherapy, photodynamic therapy, or radiation therapy. People with melanoma may also have biological therapy.

You may have a team of specialists to help plan your treatment. Your doctor may refer you to a specialist, or you may ask for a referral. Specialists who treat skin cancer include dermatologists and surgeons. Some people may also need a reconstructive or plastic surgeon.

People with advanced skin cancer may be referred to a medical oncologist or radiation oncologist. Your health care team may also include an oncology nurse, a social worker, and a registered dietitian.

You may want to ask your doctor these questions before you begin treatment:

- What is the stage of the disease? Has the cancer spread? Do any lymph nodes or other organs show signs of cancer?
- What are my treatment choices? Which do you suggest for me? Why?
- What are the expected benefits of each kind of treatment?
- What can I do to prepare for treatment?
- Will I need to stay in the hospital? If so, for how long?
- What are the risks and possible side effects of each treatment? How can side effects be managed?
- Will there be a scar? Will I need a skin graft or plastic surgery?
- What is the treatment likely to cost? Will my insurance cover it?
- How will treatment affect my normal activities?
- Would a research study (clinical trial) be a good choice for me?
- How often should I have checkups?

Source: NCI, January 11, 2011.

Because skin cancer treatment may damage healthy cells and tissues, unwanted side effects sometimes occur. Side effects depend mainly on the type and extent of the treatment. Side effects may not be the same for each person. Before treatment starts, your health care team will tell you about possible side effects and suggest ways to help you manage them.

Many skin cancers can be removed quickly and easily. But some people may need supportive care to control pain and other symptoms, to relieve the side effects of treatment, and to help them cope with the feelings that a diagnosis of cancer can bring.

You may want to talk with your doctor about taking part in a clinical trial, a research study of new treatment methods.

Surgery

In general, the surgeon will remove the cancerous growth and some normal tissue around it. This reduces the chance that cancer cells will be left in the area.

There are several methods of surgery for skin cancer. The method your doctor uses depends mainly on the type of skin cancer, the size of the cancer, and where it was found on your body. Your doctor can further describe these methods of surgery:

- **Excisional Skin Surgery:** This is a common treatment to remove any type of skin cancer. After numbing the area of skin, the surgeon removes the growth (tumor) with a scalpel. The surgeon also removes a border (a margin) of normal skin around the growth. The margin of skin is examined under a microscope to be certain that all the cancer cells have been removed. The thickness of the margin depends on the size of the tumor.

- **Mohs Surgery (Also Called Mohs Micrographic Surgery):** This method is often used for basal cell and squamous cell skin cancers. After numbing the area of skin, a specially trained surgeon shaves away thin layers of the tumor. Each layer is examined under a microscope. The surgeon continues to shave away tissue until no cancer cells can be seen under the microscope. In this way, the surgeon can remove all the cancer and only a small bit of healthy tissue. Some people will have radiation therapy after Mohs surgery to make sure all of the cancer cells are destroyed.

- **Electrodesiccation And Curettage:** This method is often used to remove a small basal cell or squamous cell skin cancer. After the doctor numbs the area to be treated, the cancer is removed with a sharp tool shaped like a spoon (called a curette). The doctor then uses a needle-shaped electrode to send an electric current into the treated area to control bleeding and kill any cancer cells that may be left. This method is usually fast and simple. It may be performed up to three times to remove all of the cancer.

- **Cryosurgery:** This method is an option for an early-stage or a very thin basal cell or squamous cell skin cancer. Cryosurgery is often used for people who are not able to have other types of surgery. The doctor applies liquid nitrogen (which is extremely cold) directly to the skin growth to freeze and kill the cancer cells. This treatment may cause swelling. It also may damage nerves, which can cause a loss of feeling in the damaged area.

For people with cancer that has spread to the lymph nodes, the surgeon may remove some or all of the nearby lymph nodes. Additional treatment may be needed after surgery.

If a large area of tissue is removed, the surgeon may do a skin graft. The doctor uses skin from another part of the body to replace the skin that was removed. After numbing the area, the surgeon removes a patch of healthy skin from another part of the body, such as the upper thigh. The patch is then used to cover the area where skin cancer was removed. If you have a skin graft, you may have to take special care of the area until it heals.

The time it takes to heal after surgery is different for each person. You may have pain for the first few days. Medicine can help control your pain. Before surgery, you should discuss the plan for pain relief with your doctor or nurse. After surgery, your doctor can adjust the plan if you need more pain relief.

Surgery nearly always leaves some type of scar. The size and color of the scar depend on the size of the cancer, the type of surgery, the color of your skin, and how your skin heals.

You may want to ask your doctor these questions before having surgery:

- What kind of surgery do you recommend for me? Why?
- Will you remove lymph nodes? Why?
- Will I need a skin graft?
- What will the scar look like? Can anything be done to help reduce the scar? Will I need plastic surgery or reconstructive surgery?
- How will I feel after surgery?
- If I have pain, how will you control it?
- Will I need to stay in the hospital? If so, for how long?
- Am I likely to have infection, swelling, blistering, or bleeding, or to get a scab where the cancer was removed?
- Will I have any long-term side effects?

Source: NCI, January 11, 2011.

For any type of surgery, including skin grafts or reconstructive surgery, follow your doctor's advice on bathing, shaving, exercise, or other activities.

Chemotherapy

Chemotherapy uses drugs to kill cancer cells. Drugs for skin cancer can be given in many ways.

Put Directly On The Skin

A cream or lotion form of chemotherapy may be used to treat very thin, early-stage basal cell or squamous cell skin cancer (Bowen disease). It may also be used if there are several small skin cancers. The doctor will show you how to apply the cream or lotion to the skin one or two times a day for several weeks.

The cream or lotion contains a drug that kills cancer cells only in the top layer of the skin:

- **Fluorouracil (Another Name Is 5-FU):** This drug is used to treat early-stage basal cell and squamous cell cancers.

- **Imiquimod:** This drug is used to treat early-stage basal cell cancer.

These drugs may cause your skin to turn red or swell. Your skin also may itch, ooze, or develop a rash. Your skin may be sore or sensitive to the sun after treatment. These skin changes usually go away after treatment is over.

A cream or lotion form of chemotherapy usually does not leave a scar. If healthy skin becomes too red or raw when the skin cancer is treated, your doctor may stop treatment.

Swallowed Or Injected

People with melanoma may receive chemotherapy by mouth or through a vein (intravenous). You may receive one or more drugs. The drugs enter the bloodstream and travel throughout the body.

If you have melanoma on an arm or leg, you may receive drugs directly into the bloodstream of that limb. The flow of blood to and from the limb is stopped for a while. This allows a high dose of drugs in the area with the melanoma. Most of the chemotherapy remains in that limb.

You may receive chemotherapy in an outpatient part of the hospital, at the doctor's office, or at home. Some people need to stay in the hospital during treatment.

The side effects depend mainly on which drugs are given and how much. Chemotherapy kills fast-growing cancer cells, but the drugs can also harm normal cells that divide rapidly:

- **Blood Cells:** When drugs lower the levels of healthy blood cells, you're more likely to get infections, bruise or bleed easily, and feel very weak and tired. Your health care team will check for low levels of blood cells. If your levels are low, your health care team may stop the chemotherapy for a while or reduce the dose of the drug. There are also medicines that can help your body make new blood cells.

- **Cells In Hair Roots:** Chemotherapy may cause hair loss. If you lose your hair, it will grow back after treatment, but the color and texture may be changed.

- **Cells That Line The Digestive Tract:** Chemotherapy can cause a poor appetite, nausea and vomiting, diarrhea, or mouth and lip sores. Your health care team can give you medicines and suggest other ways to help with these problems. They usually go away when treatment ends.

You may want to ask your doctor these questions about chemotherapy:

- Why do I need this treatment?
- Which drug or drugs will I have?
- How do the drugs work?
- Do I need to take special care when I put chemotherapy on my skin? What do I need to do? Will I be sensitive to the sun?
- When will treatment start? When will it end?
- Will I have any long-term side effects?

Source: NCI, January 11, 2011.

Photodynamic Therapy

Photodynamic therapy (PDT) uses a drug along with a special light source, such as a laser light, to kill cancer cells. PDT may be used to treat very thin, early-stage basal cell or squamous cell skin cancer (Bowen disease).

The drug is either rubbed into the skin or injected intravenously. The drug is absorbed by cancer cells. It stays in cancer cells longer than in normal cells. Several hours or days later, a special light is focused on the cancer. The drug becomes active and destroys the cancer cells.

The side effects of PDT are usually not serious. PDT may cause burning or stinging pain. It also may cause burns, swelling, or redness. It may scar healthy tissue near the growth. If you have PDT, you will need to avoid direct sunlight and bright indoor light for at least six weeks after treatment.

> You may want to ask your doctor these questions about photodynamic therapy:
>
> - Will I need to stay in the hospital while the drug is in my body?
> - Will I need to have the treatment more than once?
>
> Source: NCI, January 11, 2011.

Biological Therapy

Some people with advanced melanoma receive a drug called biological therapy. Biological therapy for melanoma is treatment that may improve the body's natural defense (immune system response) against cancer.

One drug for melanoma is interferon. It's injected intravenously (usually at a hospital or clinic) or injected under the skin (at home or in a doctor's office). Interferon can slow the growth of melanoma cells.

Another drug used for melanoma is interleukin-2. It's given intravenously. It can help the body destroy cancer cells. Interleukin-2 is usually given at the hospital.

Other drugs may be given at the same time to prevent side effects. The side effects differ with the drug used, and from person to person. Biological therapies commonly cause a rash or swelling. You may feel very tired during treatment. These drugs may also cause a headache, muscle aches, a fever, or weakness.

Radiation Therapy

Radiation therapy uses high-energy rays to kill cancer cells. The radiation comes from a large machine outside the body. It affects cells only in the treated area. You will go to a hospital or clinic several times for this treatment.

> You may want to ask your doctor these questions about biological therapy:
>
> - What is the goal of treatment?
> - When will treatment start? When will it end?
> - Will I need to stay in the hospital for treatment? If so, how long will I be in the hospital?
>
> Source: NCI, January 11, 2011.

Radiation therapy is not a common treatment for skin cancer. But it may be used for skin cancer in areas where surgery could be difficult or leave a bad scar. For example, you may have radiation therapy if you have a growth on your eyelid, ear, or nose. Radiation therapy may also be used after surgery for squamous cell carcinoma that can't be completely removed or that has spread to the lymph nodes. And it may be used for melanoma that has spread to the lymph nodes, brain, bones, or other parts of the body.

Although radiation therapy is painless, it may cause other side effects. The side effects depend mainly on the dose of radiation and the part of your body that is treated. It's common for the skin in the treated area to become red, dry, tender, and itchy. Your health care team can suggest ways to relieve the side effects of radiation therapy.

Second Opinion

Before starting treatment, you might want a second opinion from another doctor about your diagnosis and treatment plan. Some people worry that their doctor will be offended if they ask for a second opinion. Usually the opposite is true. Most doctors welcome a second opinion. And many health insurance companies will pay for a second opinion if you or your doctor requests it. Some companies require a second opinion.

If you get a second opinion, the doctor may agree with your first doctor's diagnosis and treatment plan. Or the second doctor may suggest another approach. Either way, you'll have more information and perhaps a greater sense of control. You may also feel more confident about the decisions you make, knowing that you've looked carefully at all of your options.

It may take some time and effort to gather your medical records and see another doctor. Usually it's not a problem if it takes you several weeks to get a second opinion. In most cases, the delay in starting treatment will not make treatment less effective. To make sure, you should discuss this possible delay with your doctor. Some people with skin cancer need treatment right away.

There are many ways to find a doctor for a second opinion. You can ask your doctor, a local or state medical society, or a nearby hospital or a medical school for names of specialists.

Taking Part In Cancer Research

Doctors all over the country are conducting many types of clinical trials (research studies in which people volunteer to take part). Clinical trials are designed to find out whether new treatments are safe and effective.

You may want to ask your doctor these questions about radiation therapy:

- How will I feel after treatment?
- Am I likely to have infection, swelling, blistering, or bleeding after radiation therapy?
- Will I get a scar on the treated area?
- How should I take care of the treated area?

Source: NCI, January 11, 2011.

Doctors are trying to find better ways to care for people with skin cancer. They are studying many types of treatment, such as surgery, chemotherapy, biological therapy, and combinations of treatment. For example, doctors are studying the use of a cancer treatment vaccine after surgery for people with advanced melanoma.

Even if the people in a trial do not benefit directly, they may still make an important contribution by helping doctors learn more about skin cancer and how to control it. Although clinical trials may pose some risks, doctors do all they can to protect their patients.

The National Cancer Institute (NCI) website includes a section on clinical trials at http://www.cancer.gov/clinicaltrials.

Follow-Up Care

After treatment for skin cancer, you'll need regular checkups (such as every three to six months for the first year or two). Your doctor will monitor your recovery and check for any new skin cancers. Regular checkups help ensure that any changes in your health are noted and treated if needed.

During a checkup, you'll have a physical exam. People with melanoma may have x-rays, blood tests, and scans of the chest, liver, bones, and brain.

People who have had melanoma have an increased risk of developing a new melanoma, and people with basal or squamous cell skin cancers have a risk of developing another skin cancer of any type. It's a good idea to get in a routine for checking your skin for new growths or other changes. Keep in mind that changes are not a sure sign of skin cancer. Still, you should tell your doctor about any changes right away.

Follow your doctor's advice about how to reduce your risk of developing skin cancer again.

Anyone Can Get Skin Cancer

Is it true that only people with light skin get skin cancer?

No. Anyone can get skin cancer. It's more common among people with a light (fair) skin tone, but skin cancer can affect anyone. Skin cancer can affect both men and women.

How can people with dark skin get skin cancer?

Although dark skin does not burn in the sun as easily as fair skin, everyone is at risk for skin cancer. Even people who don't burn are at risk for skin cancer. It doesn't matter whether you consider your skin light, dark, or somewhere in between. You are at risk for skin cancer. Being in the sun can damage your skin. Sunlight causes damage through ultraviolet, or UV rays, (they make up just one part of sunlight). Two parts of UV, UVA and UVB, can both cause damage to skin. Also, the sun isn't the only cause of skin cancer. There are other causes. That's why skin cancer may be found in places on the body never exposed to the sun.

Source: "Anyone Can Get Skin Cancer," National Cancer Institute, April 26, 2011.

Prevention

People with skin cancer are at risk of developing another skin cancer. Limit your time in the sun and stay away from sunlamps and tanning booths. Keep in mind that getting a tan may increase your risk of developing another skin cancer.

The best way to prevent skin cancer is to protect yourself from the sun:

- Avoid outdoor activities during the middle of the day. The sun's rays are the strongest between 10 a.m. and 4 p.m. When you must be outdoors, seek shade when you can.

- Protect yourself from the sun's rays reflected by sand, water, snow, ice, and pavement. The sun's rays can go through light clothing, windshields, windows, and clouds.

- Wear long sleeves and long pants. Tightly woven fabrics are best.

- Wear a hat with a wide brim all around that shades your face, neck, and ears. Keep in mind that baseball caps and some sun visors protect only parts of your skin.

- Wear sunglasses that absorb UV radiation to protect the skin around your eyes.

- Use sunscreen lotions with a sun protection factor (SPF) of at least 15. (Some doctors will suggest using a lotion with an SPF of at least 30.) Apply the product's recommended amount to uncovered skin 30 minutes before going outside, and apply again every two hours or after swimming or sweating.

Sunscreen lotions may help prevent some skin cancers. It's important to use a broad-spectrum sunscreen lotion that filters both UVB and UVA radiation. But you still need to avoid the sun during the middle of the day and wear clothing to protect your skin.

How To Check Your Skin

Your doctor or nurse may suggest that you do a regular skin self-exam to check for the development of a new skin cancer.

The best time to do this exam is after a shower or bath. Check your skin in a room with plenty of light. Use a full-length mirror and a hand-held mirror.

It's best to begin by learning where your birthmarks, moles, and other marks are and their usual look and feel.

Check for anything new, including the following:

- A new mole (that looks different from your other moles)
- A new red or darker color flaky patch that may be a little raised
- A new flesh-colored firm bump
- A change in the size, shape, color, or feel of a mole
- A sore that doesn't heal

Check yourself from head to toe in the following way:

- Look at your face, neck, ears, and scalp. You may want to use a comb or a blow dryer to move your hair so that you can see better. You also may want to have a relative or friend check through your hair. It may be hard to check your scalp by yourself.
- Look at the front and back of your body in the mirror. Then, raise your arms and look at your left and right sides.
- Bend your elbows. Look carefully at your fingernails, palms, forearms (including the undersides), and upper arms.
- Examine the back, front, and sides of your legs. Also look around your genital area and between your buttocks.

- Sit and closely examine your feet, including your toenails, your soles, and the spaces between your toes.

By checking your skin regularly, you'll learn what is normal for you. It may be helpful to record the dates of your skin exams and to write notes about the way your skin looks. If your doctor has taken photos of your skin, you can compare your skin to the photos to help check for changes. If you find anything unusual, see your doctor.

Sources Of Support

Learning that you have skin cancer can change your life and the lives of those close to you. These changes can be hard to handle. It's normal for you, your family, and your friends to need help coping with the feelings that such a diagnosis can bring.

Concerns about treatments and managing side effects, hospital stays, and medical bills are common. You may also worry about caring for your family, keeping your job, or continuing daily activities.

Here's where you can go for support:

- Doctors, nurses, and other members of your health care team can answer questions about treatment, working, or other activities.

- Social workers, counselors, or members of the clergy can be helpful if you want to talk about your feelings or concerns. Often, social workers can suggest resources for financial aid, transportation, home care, or emotional support.

- Support groups also can help. In these groups, people with skin cancer or their family members meet with other patients or their families to share what they have learned about coping with the disease and the effects of treatment. Groups may offer support in person, over the telephone, or on the Internet. You may want to talk with a member of your health care team about finding a support group

- NCI's Cancer Information Service at 1-800-4-CANCER (1-800-422-6237) and at LiveHelp (http://www.cancer.gov/livehelp) can help you locate programs, services, and NCI publications. They can send you a list of organizations that offer services to people with cancer.

Chapter 33

Moles, Skin Tags, Lentigines, And Seborrheic Keratoses

There are several skin lesions that are very common and almost always benign (non-cancerous). These conditions include moles, freckles, skin tags, lentigines, and seborrheic keratoses.

What is a mole?

Moles are growths on the skin that are usually pink or brown. Moles can appear anywhere on the skin, alone or in groups.

Most moles appear in early childhood and during the first 20 years of a person's life. Some moles might not appear until later in life. It is normal to have between 10 and 40 moles by adulthood.

As the years pass, moles usually change slowly, becoming raised and lighter in color. Often, hairs develop on the mole. Some moles will not change at all, while others will slowly disappear over time.

What causes a mole?

Moles occur when cells in the skin grow in a cluster instead of being spread throughout the skin. These cells are called melanocytes, and they make the pigment that gives skin its natural color. Moles might darken after exposure to the sun, during the teen years, and during pregnancy.

About This Chapter: From "Moles, Freckles, Skin Tags, Benign Lentigines, and Seborrheic Keratoses," © 2013 The Cleveland Clinic Foundation, 9500 Euclid Avenue, Cleveland, OH 44195. All rights reserved. Reprinted with permission. Additional information is available from the Cleveland Clinic Health Information Center, 216-444-3771, toll-free 800-223-2273 extension 43771, or at http://my.clevelandclinic.org/health.

What should I look for when examining my moles?

Most moles are benign. The only moles that are of medical concern are those that look different than other existing moles or those that first appear after age 20. If you notice changes in a mole's color, height, size, or shape, you should have a dermatologist (skin doctor) evaluate it. You also should have moles checked if they bleed, ooze, itch, appear scaly, or become tender or painful.

Examine your skin monthly with a mirror or ask someone to help you. Pay special attention to areas of your skin that are often exposed to the sun, such as the hands, arms, chest, neck, face, and ears.

If your moles do not change over time, there is little reason for concern. If you see any signs of change in an existing mole, if you have a new mole, or if you want a mole to be removed for cosmetic reasons, talk to your dermatologist.

The following ABCDEs are important signs of moles that could be cancerous. If a mole displays any of the signs listed below, have it checked immediately by a dermatologist:

- **A**symmetry: One half of the mole does not match the other half.

- **B**order: The border or edges of the mole are ragged, blurred, or irregular.

- **C**olor: The color of the mole is not the same throughout or has shades of tan, brown, black, blue, white, or red.

- **D**iameter: The diameter of a mole is larger than the eraser of a pencil (6 millimeters).

- **E**levation/Evolution: A mole appears elevated, or raised, from the skin. Are the moles changing over time?

Melanoma is a form of skin cancer. The most common location for melanoma in men is the back; in women, it is the lower leg. Melanoma is the most common cancer in women ages 25 to 29.

What are the different types of moles?

Congenital nevi are moles that are present at birth. Congenital nevi occur in about one in 100 people. These moles might be more likely to develop into melanoma than moles that appear after birth. If the mole is more than 8 inches in diameter, it poses more risk of becoming cancerous.

Dysplastic nevi are moles that are larger than average (larger than a pencil eraser) and irregular in shape. They tend to have uneven color with dark brown centers and lighter, uneven edges. These moles tend to be hereditary. People with dysplastic nevi might have more than 100 moles and have a greater chance of developing malignant (cancerous) melanoma. Any changes in the mole should be checked by a dermatologist to detect skin cancer.

How are moles treated?

If a dermatologist believes the mole needs to be evaluated further or removed entirely, he or she will first take a biopsy (small tissue sample of the mole) to examine thin sections of the tissue under a microscope. This is a simple procedure. (If the dermatologist thinks the mole might be cancerous, cutting through the mole will not cause the cancer to spread.)

If the mole is found to be cancerous, the dermatologist will remove the entire mole by cutting out the entire mole and a rim of normal skin around it, and stitching the wound closed.

What is a skin tag?

A skin tag is a small flap of tissue that hangs off the skin by a connecting stalk. Skin tags are benign and are not dangerous. They are usually found on the neck, chest, back, armpits, under the breasts, or in the groin area. Skin tags appear most often in women, especially with weight gain, and in middle-aged and elderly people.

Skin tags usually don't cause any pain. However, they can become irritated if anything such as clothing or jewelry rubs on them.

How are skin tags treated?

Your dermatologist can remove a skin tag by cutting it off with a scalpel or scissors, with cryotherapy (freezing it off), or with electrosurgery (burning with an electric current).

What is a lentigo?

A lentigo (plural: lentigines) is a spot on the skin that is darker (usually brown) than the surrounding skin. Lentigines are more common among Caucasian patients, especially those with fair skin.

What are the causes of lentigines?

Exposure to the sun seems to be the major cause of lentigines. Lentigines most often appear on parts of the body that get the most sun, including the face and hands. Some lentigines might be caused by genetics (family history) or by medical procedures such as radiation therapy.

How are lentigines treated?

There are several methods for treating lentigines:

- Cryotherapy (freezing it off)

- Laser surgery
- Creams that are applied to the skin (These include retinoids and bleaching agents.)

Can lentigines be prevented?

The best way to prevent lentigines is to stay out of the sun as much as possible. Use sunscreen when outdoors, and avoid using a tanning bed to get a suntan.

What are freckles?

Freckles are small brown spots usually found on the face and arms. Freckles are extremely common and are not a health threat. They are more often seen in the summer, especially among lighter-skinned people and people with light or red hair. Both men and women get freckles at an equal rate.

What causes freckles?

Causes of freckles include genetics, diseases (such as xeroderma pigmentosum, a rare disease that causes an increased sensitivity to ultraviolet light, such as the sun), and exposure to the sun.

What is the treatment for freckles?

Since freckles are almost always harmless, there really is no need to treat them. As with many skin conditions, it's best to avoid the sun as much as possible, or use a sunscreen. This is especially important because people who freckle easily (such as lighter-skinned people) are more likely to develop skin cancer.

If you feel that your freckles are a problem or you don't like the way they look, you can cover them up with makeup.

What are seborrheic keratoses?

Seborrheic keratoses are brown or black growths usually found on the chest and back, as well as on the head. They originate from cells called keratinocytes. As they develop, seborrheic keratoses take on a warty appearance.

What causes seborrheic keratoses?

The cause of seborrheic keratoses is unknown. They are seen more often as people get older. They do not lead to skin cancer.

How are seborrheic keratoses treated?

Seborrheic keratoses are benign and are not contagious. Therefore, they don't need to be treated.

If you decide to have seborrheic keratoses removed because you don't like the way they look, or because they are chronically irritated by clothing, methods for removing them include cutting them off, cryotherapy, and electrosurgery.

Can seborrheic keratoses be prevented?

Seborrheic keratoses can't be prevented.

Chapter 34

Pruritus (Itching)

Introduction

Itching is an unpleasant sensation that compels a person to scratch the affected area. It is a common symptom but occasionally may be severe and frustrating. The medical name for itching is pruritus.

Itching can affect any area of the body. It can either be:

- **Generalized:** Where itching occurs over the whole body

- **Localized:** Where itching only occurs in a particular area

Sometimes, there is a rash or a spot where the itching occurs.

Common Causes Of Itching

Itching can be caused by a number of different conditions. For example:

- A skin condition, such as eczema

- An allergy or skin reaction

- A parasitic infestation, such as scabies

- Insect bites and insect stings

- A fungal infection, such as athlete's foot or thrush

- A systemic condition (one that affects the whole body), such as an overactive thyroid gland (hyperthyroidism)

- Hormonal changes during pregnancy or the menopause

Things You Can Do

In many cases, treating the underlying condition will ease the itching. However, there are things you can do to relieve itching, including:

- Using a cold compress, such as a flannel

- Applying calamine lotion to the affect area

- Using unperfumed personal hygiene products

- Bathing in cool water

- Not wearing clothes that irritate your skin, such as wool and man-made fabrics

- Keeping skin moist

There are also medicines such as antihistamines and steroid creams that may help to relieve the symptoms of itching caused by certain skin conditions.

How To Avoid Scratching

Scratching can damage the skin and irritate it further, which can make it painful and itch more. The following might help you avoid scratching:

- Rub or press the affected area with your palm.
- Keep the itchy skin moist with an emollient, which makes scratching less damaging to the skin.

It's not easy to avoid scratching so keep your nails short and clean. Nails should be filed not clipped; clipped nails can often have jagged edges that could damage your skin when scratching.

When To See Your Doctor

Many cases of itching will get better over a short period of time. However, it is important to visit your doctor if your itching is not improving or is affecting your quality of life.

You should see your doctor if your itching is:

- Severe

- Lasts for a long time

- Keeps coming back

- Associated with other symptoms, such as breathing problems, skin inflammation, or jaundice (yellowing of the skin and eyes)

Also visit your doctor as soon as possible if your entire body itches and there is no obvious cause. It could be a symptom of a more serious condition.

Your doctor may carry out tests to determine the cause of the itching, such as:

- A skin scraping: The affected area of skin is scraped to obtain a sample, which can be analyzed to help diagnose a skin condition.

- A vaginal or penile swab if a yeast infection is suspected; a small plastic rod with a cotton ball on one end will be used to obtain the sample.

- A blood test to see if the cause is an underlying disease, such as diabetes, thyroid, or kidney disease.

- A biopsy: The area is numbed and a tissue sample is removed for analysis.

Causes Of Itching

There are many different possible causes of itching. For example, itching can be a symptom of:

- A skin condition, such as eczema

- An allergy—for example, to nickel (a metal often used to make costume jewelry)

- Insect bites, or scabies (a contagious skin condition where tiny mites burrow into the skin)

- Fungal infections, such as athlete's foot and female thrush or male thrush (a fungal infection that affects the male and female genitals)

- Certain chronic (long-term) conditions, such as liver disease

- Hormonal changes in the body, such as during the menopause (when a woman's periods stop, usually at around 52 years of age)

Skin Conditions

Skin conditions that can cause itching include:

- **Dry Skin**

- **Eczema:** A chronic (long-term) condition where the skin is dry, red, flaky, and itchy
- **Contact Dermatitis:** A condition where the skin becomes inflamed
- **Urticaria:** Also known as hives, welts, or nettle rash, urticaria is triggered by an allergen, such as food or latex, and causes a raised, red, itchy rash to develop
- **Lichen Planus:** An itchy, non-infectious rash of unknown cause
- **Psoriasis:** A non-infectious skin condition that causes red, flaky, crusty patches of skin and silvery scales
- **Dandruff:** A common, non-contagious skin condition that affects the scalp
- **Folliculitis:** A skin condition caused by inflamed hair follicles
- **Prurigo:** Small blisters (fluid-filled swellings) that are very itchy

Allergies And Skin Reactions

Itching is sometimes caused by environmental factors, such as:

- Cosmetics
- Dyes or coatings on fabrics
- Contact with certain metals, such as nickel
- Contact with the juices of certain plants or stinging plants
- An allergy to certain foods or types of medication (for example, aspirin and a group of medicines called opioids)
- Prickly heat: An itchy rash that appears in hot, humid weather conditions
- Sunburn: Skin damage caused by exposure to ultraviolet (UV) rays

Parasites And Insects

Itching can also be caused by the following pests:

- The scabies mite, which burrows into the skin and causes a skin condition called scabies
- Head lice, pubic lice, or body lice
- Insect bites and stings, such as bees, wasps, mosquitoes, fleas, and bedbugs

Infections

Itching may also be a symptom of an infection, such as:

- Chickenpox or another viral infection

- A fungal infection, such as athlete's foot, which causes itching in between the toes, jock itch which affects the groin, and ringworm, a contagious condition that causes a ring-like red rash to develop on the body

- A yeast infection, such as female thrush or male thrush, which can cause itching in and around the genitals

Fungal and yeast infections tend to cause itching in a specific area of the body. But in untreated cases, or cases that do not respond well to treatment, itching may become generalized.

Systemic Conditions

Systemic conditions are conditions that affect the entire body. Sometimes, itching can be a symptom of systemic conditions, such as:

- An overactive thyroid or underactive thyroid—the thyroid gland is found in the neck; it produces hormones to help control the body's growth and metabolism (the process of turning food into energy)

- Liver-related conditions, such as primary biliary cirrhosis, liver cancer, pancreatic cancer, and hepatitis

- Long-standing kidney failure

- Leukemia: Cancer of the blood

- Some types of cancers, such as breast, lung, and prostate cancer

- Hodgkin lymphoma: Cancer of the lymphatic system, which is a series of glands (or nodes) spread throughout your body that produce many of the specialized cells needed by your immune system

Itchy Bottom

Itchy bottom, also known as *pruritus ani,* is a common condition where there is a very strong urge to scratch the skin around the anus (back passage). It can have a number of different causes, including:

- **Threadworms:** Small worm parasites that infect the bowels of humans
- **Hemorrhoids (Piles):** Enlarged and swollen blood vessels in or around the lower rectum or anus

Pregnancy And Menopause

In women, itching can sometimes be caused by hormonal changes.

Pregnancy

Itching often affects pregnant women and usually disappears after the birth. A number of skin conditions can develop during pregnancy and cause itchy skin. They include:

- **Pruritic Urticarial Papules And Plaques Of Pregnancy (PUPPP):** A common skin condition during pregnancy that causes itchy, red, raised bumps that appear on the thighs and abdomen (tummy)

- **Prurigo Gestationis:** A skin rash that appears as red, itchy dots and mainly affects the arms, legs, and torso

- **Obstetric Cholestasis:** A rare disorder that affects the liver during pregnancy and causes itching of the skin without a skin rash

Eczema and psoriasis are also skin conditions that pregnant women may experience.

Seek advice from your midwife or doctor if you have itching or any unusual skin rashes during your pregnancy.

Menopause

Itching is also a common symptom of the menopause, which is where a woman's periods stop, at around 52 years of age, as a result of hormonal changes. Changes in the levels of hormones, such as estrogen, that occur during the menopause are thought to be responsible for the itching.

Treatment

The type of treatment you receive for itching will depend on the cause.

If you are referred for further investigations, there are things you can do yourself to give you some relief.

Using a cold compress such as damp flannel, or applying calamine lotion to the affected area may help relieve your itching.

Bathing

When bathing or showering you should:

- Use cool or lukewarm water (not hot).

- Avoid using perfumed soap, shower gel or deodorants; unperfumed lotions or aqueous cream are available from your pharmacist.

- Use unperfumed moisturizing lotions and emollients after bathing or showering to help prevent your skin becoming too dry.

Clothing And Fabric

Regarding clothing and bed linen, you should:

- Avoid wearing clothes that irritate your skin, such as wool and some fabrics.

- Wear cotton whenever possible.

- Avoid tight-fitting clothes.

- Use mild laundry detergent that will not irritate your skin.

- Use cool, light, loose bedclothes.

Medication

With regard to medication, you can use:

- An oily moisturizer or emollient if your skin is dry or flaky

- Mild steroid cream (for no longer than seven days) for localized, inflamed, itchy areas—hydrocortisone cream is available from pharmacies over the counter, or your doctor can prescribe a steroid cream for you

- Antihistamine tablets to help control allergic reactions and help break the itch-scratch cycle—consult your doctor before using these because they are not suitable for all cases of itching

---

Vulval Itching

If you have itching around the outside of your vagina, your GP [health care provider] will treat the underlying cause. This could be:

- A yeast infection, such as vaginal thrush
- Contact dermatitis, sometimes caused by excessive washing or perfumed hygiene products
- A skin condition

Your doctor may prescribe emollients or antihistamines to help relieve the itching.

Antihistamine tablets may also make you feel drowsy therefore it's important you do not drive, use power tools or heavy machinery while taking them.

Some antidepressants such as paroxetine or sertraline can help relieve itching (if your doctor prescribes these, it does not mean you are depressed).

If you have itching in hairy areas, such as your scalp, lotions can be prescribed specifically for these areas, rather than using sticky creams.

Chapter 35

Psoriasis

Facts About Psoriasis

What Is Psoriasis?

Psoriasis is a genetic skin disease associated with the immune system. Your immune system causes your skin cells to reproduce too quickly. A normal skin cell matures and falls off the body's surface in 28 to 30 days. However, skin affected by psoriasis takes only three to four days to mature and move to the surface. Instead of falling off (shedding), the cells pile up and form lesions. The skin also becomes very red due to increased blood flow.

Is Psoriasis Contagious?

Psoriasis is not contagious. It is not something you can "catch" or "pass on." The lesions may not look good, but they are not infections or open wounds. People with psoriasis pose no threat to the health or safety of others.

Who Gets Psoriasis?

The disease affects as many as 7.5 million people in the United States. Ordinarily, people have their first outbreak between the ages of 15 and 35, but it can appear at any age. Approximately one-third of those who get psoriasis are under 20 years old when the disease first surfaces.

What Causes Psoriasis?

No one knows exactly what causes psoriasis, but it has a genetic component. Most researchers agree that the immune system is mistakenly triggered, which speeds up the growth cycle of skin cells. A person can have the genes for psoriasis without having the disease on their skin. Genes may be passed through several generations of a family before someone encounters the "right" mix of genes and environmental factors that lead to the development of psoriasis.

Is There A Cure?

Currently, there is no cure for psoriasis. However, there is hope for a cure. Researchers are studying psoriasis more than ever before. They understand much more about its genetic causes and how it involves the immune system. The National Psoriasis Foundation and the federal government are promoting and funding research to find the cause and cure for psoriasis.

Are There Different Types Of Psoriasis?

There are five forms of psoriasis:

- Plaque [plak] psoriasis: The most common form, characterized by inflamed skin lesions topped with white scales.
- Guttate [GUH-tate]: Characterized by small dot-like lesions.
- Pustular [PUHS-choo-ler]: Characterized by pus-filled, blister-like lesions, and intense scaling.
- Inverse: Characterized by intense inflammation in the folds of the skin.
- Erythrodermic [eh-REETH-ro-der-mik]: Characterized by intense shedding and redness of the skin. If this rare form develops, see a doctor immediately.

Approximately 10 percent to 30 percent of people with psoriasis will develop psoriatic arthritis. This form of arthritis is similar to rheumatoid arthritis. It can develop at any time, but for most people it appears between the ages of 30 and 50. In psoriatic arthritis, the joints and the soft tissue around them become inflamed and stiff. Psoriatic arthritis can affect the fingers and toes and may involve the neck, lower back, knees, and ankles. Having psoriasis does not guarantee that you will eventually develop psoriatic arthritis.

How Do I Treat It?

Psoriasis treatments work by slowing skin cell reproduction. Some help remove scale. Others help soothe itchy or uncomfortable skin. All psoriasis medications are effective in clearing lesions, but not all people with psoriasis react the same way to medications. It may require experimentation to see which treatments work for you.

Seeing The Dermatologist

Most likely, you will be treated by a dermatologist. Dermatologists are doctors who specialize in skin care and diseases. They receive training to help keep skin healthy and to treat skin problems. Depending on how much information your dermatologist has about you, they may do the following things during your dermatology appointment:

- Ask you about yourself, you skin problem, and your concerns. This is a good time to tell the doctor about any itching, burning, or redness on your skin.

- Perform a physical exam. This is when the doctor will look very closely at your skin.

- Test for anything that relates to the problem. This may include taking a sample of tissue, so that the doctor can determine what is causing the irritation.

- Explain the condition, treatment options, and side effects of the medicine. You or your guardian may ask the doctor more questions about the treatments and side effects.

- Tell your guardian about the cost and time of the treatment. You may need to return for more visits to the dermatologist. Sometimes, most of the treatment can be done at home to get rid of the lesions.

Treatments For Psoriasis

There are three basic categories of psoriasis treatment:

- Topical treatments like creams and ointments are used on the areas of skin that have psoriasis plaques.

- Light therapy (ultraviolet light A and B or UVA and UVB) works by exposing the skin to light waves, sometimes over the whole body and sometimes only on affected areas, like hands and feet.

- Systemic medications are medications taken by mouth or injected into the muscle.

Choosing A Treatment

Doctors select treatments according to the type and severity of the psoriasis, the areas of the skin affected, your age, and past medical history. Some of the treatments available for adults are used less often for teenagers because of the possibility of long-term or delayed side effects. Long-term effects on childbearing potential are important considerations for teenage girls.

Your Role In Treatment

Your overall goal is to gain control of your psoriasis and manage it. You'll need to work closely with your parents and doctor to understand your treatment options and to be sure you understand exactly how to follow the treatment directions. Half of all patients with a treatment prescribed by a doctor do not follow through as directed and, therefore, don't give the medication a fair chance to work.

Psoriasis patients report that the more they know about their treatment and take part in managing their treatment, the better prepared they are to develop reasonable expectations about treatment. They know what to expect and are more likely to use their medications correctly.

Discussing Treatment With Your Doctor

Here are some questions you can ask your doctor when you are deciding which treatment to use for your psoriasis:

- How long has this treatment been used for psoriasis?

- What are the potential benefits of the treatment?

- What percent of people improve on this therapy?

- How quickly will it work?

- How long will it work?

- What are the common side effects of the therapy?

- Will tests be required to monitor the side effects? If so, what kinds of tests and how often will I need them?

- Will the side effects go away if I stop the medicine?

- Can I stop this treatment suddenly or do I need to quit gradually?

- What are the other options?

- What if this treatment fails?

Chapter 36

Pyogenic Granuloma And Pityriasis Rosea

Pyogenic Granuloma

Pyogenic granuloma is a relatively common skin growth. It is usually a small red, oozing and bleeding bump that looks like raw hamburger meat. It often seems to follows a minor injury and grows rapidly over a period of a few weeks to an average size of a half an inch. The head, neck, upper trunk, and hands and feet are the most common sites.

Pyogenic granuloma can occur at any age, but is least common in the very young and the very old. It is seen most often in children, pregnant women ("pregnancy tumor"), and those taking the drugs Indinavir, Soriatane, Accutane, and oral contraceptives.

Pyogenic granulomas are always benign growths. Still there is always a concern that they could be cancerous, and rarely a cancer can mimic pyogenic granuloma. A sample is usually obtained for biopsy analysis. This is particularly important since as many as half of treated cases will recur (grow back) and need a second treatment.

Those that appear on the upper back in young adults are more prone to recur. At times multiple smaller pyogenic granulomas form following a treatment (these are known as "satellites"). It appears that pieces of pyogenic granuloma may spread though local blood vessels. Pyogenic granulomas in pregnant women may go away after delivery on their own, and sometimes waiting is the best strategy in those cases.

Most pyogenic granulomas are scraped off with an instrument called a curette and lightly cauterized to decrease the chance they will re-grow. An injection of local anesthesia is required (lidocaine is used—similar to Novocaine). Some doctors prefer to treat with chemicals (TCA, podophyllin, phenol, silver nitrate). Laser surgery can also be done but has not been proven to be superior. The highest cure rates are obtained when the growth is removed by full thickness surgical excision, and closed with stitches.

Pityriasis Rosea

Pityriasis rosea is a common skin disease. It appears as a rash that can last from several weeks to several months. The way the rash looks may differ from person to person. It most often develops in the spring and the fall, and seems to favor adolescents and young adults. Pityriasis rosea is uncommon in those over 60 years old. It may last months longer when it occurs in this age group. Usually there are no permanent marks as a result of this disease, although some darker-skinned persons may develop long-lasting flat brown spots.

The skin rash follows a very distinctive pattern. In three-fourths of the cases, a single, isolated, oval scaly patch (the "herald patch") appears on the body, particularly on the trunk, upper arms, neck, or thighs. Often, the herald patch is mistaken for ringworm (*tinea corporis*) or eczema. Within a week or two more pink patches will occur on the body and on the arms and legs. These patches often form a pattern over the back resembling the outline of an evergreen tree with dropping branches. Patches may also appear on the neck and, rarely, on the face. These spots usually are smaller than the herald patch. The rash begins to heal after 2–4 weeks and is usually gone by 6–14.

Sometimes the disease can cause a more severe skin reaction. Some patients with this disease will have some itching that can be severe, especially when the patient becomes overheated. Occasionally there may be other symptoms, including tiredness and aching. The rash usually fades and disappears within six weeks but can sometimes last much longer. Physical activity, like jogging or running, or bathing in hot water may cause the rash to temporarily worsen or reappear. In some cases, the patches will reappear up to several weeks after the first episode. This can continue for many months.

The cause is unproven. It definitely is not caused by a fungus or bacterial infection. It also is not due to any known type of allergic reaction. This condition is not a sign of any type of internal disease. Since it is neither contagious nor sexually transmitted, there is no reason to avoid close or intimate contact when one has this eruption.

There is some evidence that it is a relapse of human herpes virus type 7 (HH7) infection, as this virus has been isolated from blood, skin lesions, and white blood cells (lymphocytes) of pityriasis rosea patients. In other people HH7 is only found in the lymphocytes. This virus infects most of us as children, and we develop immunity to it. This is the reason it is so very uncommon for other members of the same household to come down with pityriasis rosea at the same time.

A dermatologist can usually diagnose the condition quickly with an examination, but at times the diagnosis is more difficult. The numbers and sizes of the spots can vary and occasionally the rash can be found in an unusual location, such as the lower body or on the face. When there is no "herald" patch, reactions to medications, infection with fungus or syphilis (a type of VD), or other skin diseases may resemble this rash. The dermatologist may order blood tests, skin scrapings or even may take a biopsy from one of the spots to examine under a microscope to reach a diagnosis.

Treatment may include external and internal medications for itching. Aveeno oatmeal baths, anti-itch medicated lotions, and steroid creams may be prescribed to combat the rash. Lukewarm, rather than hot, baths may be suggested. Strenuous activity, which could aggravate the rash, should be discouraged. Ultraviolet light treatments given under the supervision of a dermatologist may be helpful. Recently, both the antiviral drug Famvir and the antibiotic erythromycin have been claimed to produce healing in one to two weeks. For severe cases a few days of oral anti-inflammatory medications such as prednisone may be necessary to promote healing. For mild cases, no treatment is required as this disease is not a dangerous skin condition.

Chapter 37

Rosacea

Rosacea, or acne rosacea, is a skin disorder leading to redness and pimples on the nose, forehead, cheekbones, and chin. The inflamed pimples and redness of rosacea can look a great deal like acne, but blackheads are almost never present. It is a fairly common disorder with about one in every twenty Americans is afflicted with it. Rosacea is most common in white women between the ages of 30 and 60. When it occurs in men, it tends to be more severe and may eventually cause the nose to become red and enlarged (rhinophyma). Fair-skinned individuals and people who flush easily seem to be more susceptible to this condition.

Rosacea becomes progressively worse in many of those affected. The real cause of rosacea is now thought to be a tendency to flush and blush in a person with sun damage. Sun damages the supporting fibers of the small blood vessels just under the surface of the skin, allowing the vessels to stretch out (become permanently dilated). The damaged blood vessels leak fluid when flushing occurs, resulting in blotchy red areas. Swelling occurs, but is not usually so prominent to be very visible. The first sign most people see are small red pimples and pustules (pus-filled whiteheads). The redness can come and go and may be tender, inflamed, and sensitive to the touch. Later, the skin tissue can swell and thicken. Eventually the redness and swelling can become permanent.

Eventually the capillaries become visible through the skin's surface; these are called telangiectasis. They often start on the sides of the nose. In a fair, delicate skin predisposed to rosacea, anything that makes one flush will promote rosacea and telangiectasis. A person's lifestyle and habits can be the skin's worst enemy. The more blood vessels one has near the surface of the skin, the more one is likely to flush and stay flushed.

About This Chapter: From "Rosacea," © 2013 American Osteopathic College of Dermatology (www.aocd.org). All rights reserved. Reprinted with permission.

Flushing triggers include a steady diet of hot beverages, spicy food, alcohol (either topically applied or drinking in excess), excessive prescription steroids, physical and mental stress, extremes of weather, harsh soaps, exfoliating creams, and hot baths. Controlling the flushing can allow one to control the rosacea, sometimes without using medication. Unfortunately, what aggravates one person's rosacea may have no effect on another's.

Rosacea can affect the eyes. How severely rosacea affects the eye is not related to how severe the facial rosacea is. Symptoms that suggest ocular (eye) rosacea include a feeling of dryness and grittiness in the eyes and inflamed bumps (chalazions) on the lids. The eyelashes may develop scales and crusts, often misdiagnosed as seborrheic dermatitis. A persistent burning feeling, red eyes and light sensitivity suggest the more severe problem of rosacea keratitis. This rare complication can lead to with blindness without treatment. All patients with significant symptoms of ocular rosacea should be seen by an ophthalmologist for a thorough examination.

Telangiectasias (broken blood vessels) can be treated with electrocautery (burning the vessels with an electric needle). It gives just the right result for many people and is less expensive and more available than lasers. If a person has rhinophyma from the disorder, a laser can shave away excess tissue to restore a smoother appearance to the skin.

Treatment includes avoidance of anything that makes one flush and known precipitants of flare-ups. Overheating—whether due to direct sun, excess clothing, hot foods—is uniformly a problem. Avoid hot showers, saunas, excessively warm environments, and extremes of weather (strong winds, cold, humidity).

Foods are more inconsistent triggers, and most bother no more than one-third of rosacea patients. These include fermented products high in histamine (vinegar, yogurt, sour cream, dry cheeses, soy sauce, yeast extract), certain vegetables and fruits (eggplant, avocados, spinach, broad-leaf beans and pods, including lima, navy or pea, citrus fruits, tomatoes, bananas, red plums, raisins or figs), spicy hot food, chocolate, vanilla, and liver. Other factors include prescription medications (vasodilators, topical steroids) alcohol (red wine, beer, bourbon, gin, vodka, or champagne), menopausal flushing, chronic coughing, and emotional stress and anxiety.

Treatment will control rosacea in most cases. It should be possible to control symptoms and keep rosacea from getting worse. Rosacea comes back in most of the patients in weeks to months of stopping treatment unless all trigger factors have been stopped.

The most effective treatments are oral tetracycline and similar antibiotics and low-dose oral Accutane. Mild cases can be controlled by gels or creams such as Metrogel, Cleocin-T, Azelex, or sulfa. Often, full doses of pills are needed only for a short while. Maintenance treatment can be intermittent doses or just topical creams. For rosacea of the eyes, warm compresses to lids (hot towel) for five minutes twice a day, liquefies the oil in the gland ducts—can be very helpful.

Makeup can be an effective aid in rosacea, will not make it worse, and even some male rosacea sufferers use a bit. A slightly more olive color than usual helps to hide the redness. For some women, hormone replacement pills may be given to reduce menopausal hot flashes. Many advances have been made in recent years. Regular visits are advised for most rosacea patients.

Chapter 38

Scleroderma

Localized Scleroderma

What Is Localized Scleroderma?

Scleroderma means "hard skin." Children with localized scleroderma often have involvement of the tissues below the skin, including muscle and bone. Besides the skin hardening, there can be changes in skin color and texture, and the underlying tissues may fail to grow normally. Localized scleroderma can occur in several different forms, including linear scleroderma (where the lesion appears as a line or streak) and circumscribed morphea (where the lesion appears as a roundish lesion). Most patients have the disease on just one part or side of their body. Early on, some lesions may have a red or purplish color that may be limited to the lesion border. Others may have a white or waxy appearance and feel hard.

Fast Facts

- In children, localized scleroderma is more common and less severe than the generalized form of scleroderma, which is also called systemic sclerosis and severely affects internal organs.

- Scleroderma can cause growth and joint problems in children.

- There is no known cure, but treatments can control the disease or reduce associated problems.

About This Chapter: From "Localized Scleroderma," and "Scleroderma (Also Known As Systemic Sclerosis)," © 2012 American College of Rheumatology (www.rheumatology.org). All rights reserved. Reprinted with permission. "Localized Scleroderma" was written by Suzanne Li, M.D,. Ph.D., Francesco Zulian, M.D., and Thuy Beam, R.N.

Who Gets Localized Scleroderma?

Localized scleroderma can occur at any age and in any race, but is more common in Caucasians. Most patients who develop scleroderma are female. Environmental factors, such as trauma, infections, or drug or chemical exposure, may play a role, but not for most patients. The disease is not contagious. The disease is not passed on directly from parent to child by any one gene, though certain genes may make a child more likely to develop localized scleroderma.

Localized scleroderma is a rare disease, and the exact number of patients with this disease is not known. The best estimate is that 50 children out of every 100,000 will develop localized scleroderma.

What Causes Localized Scleroderma?

Localized scleroderma is an autoimmune disease in which the immune system causes inflammation in the skin. The inflammation can trigger connective tissue cells to produce too much collagen, a fibrous protein that is a major part of many tissues. Excess collagen can lead to fibrosis, which is like scarring.

How Is Localized Scleroderma Diagnosed?

Scleroderma usually is diagnosed by a rheumatologist or dermatologist based on the patient's history and physical examination. There are no specific laboratory studies to diagnose localized scleroderma, but tests often are done to evaluate level of inflammation and problems related to localized scleroderma, and to make sure the patient does not have another condition. A skin biopsy may be done to confirm the diagnosis.

How Is Localized Scleroderma Treated?

Treatment varies depending on the patient's disease activity, lesion location and extent, and whether there are related problems. Careful clinical evaluation is the primary method for monitoring scleroderma. X-rays and computerized tomography (CT) scans are used to look at bone abnormalities. Thermography can detect differences in skin temperature between the lesion and normal tissue. Ultrasound and magnetic resonance imaging (MRI) can aid soft tissue assessment.

Current treatment is focused on controlling inflammation, as this decreases the risk of serious problems such as differences in limb length, areas of sunken skin on the face, limited joint movement, and an internal organ problem. Patients with linear scleroderma, lesions on the head, deep lesions, or widespread disease, are usually treated with systemic medications that suppress the immune system. These medicines include methotrexate, which is given by injection or taken by mouth once a week, and corticosteroids, which is taken by mouth (prednisone) or given by infusion (intravenous methylprednisolone). A recent randomized clinical trial showed that methotrexate was better than placebo at maintaining disease control after initial corticosteroid treatment. Other immunosuppressive medicines include mycophenolate mofetil, cyclosporine, and tacrolimus. More work is needed to determine the best therapy for localized scleroderma. Immunosuppressive medicines can increase a patient's risk for developing an infection and have other possible side effects; these will be reviewed by your doctor.

For patients with mild superficial disease, topical medications often are used to control the inflammation and soften the skin. These medications include corticosteroids, calcipotriene, tacrolimus, pimecrolimus, and imiquimod. Moisturizers may help protect and soften the skin.

Phototherapy has been used to treat patients with widespread, superficial disease. Both UVB and UVA have been reported to help. More study is needed to evaluate the potential side effects from exposing children to large amounts of ultraviolet light.

Physical and occupational therapy to improve strength and function is important for patients with muscle weakness, limb length differences, and limited joint movement.

Surgery is not recommended during treatment of active disease. Surgery may be needed for patients with severe pain or limitation, and can improve the appearance of patients with severe facial lesions. However, because the skin is abnormal there can be poor wound healing, and surgery may trigger a flare of disease in some cases. Cosmetic makeup can be used to make the lesions less noticeable.

There is no known cure for localized scleroderma. The disease can stop on its own (remission), but the timing of this varies. Circumscribed morphea lesions that do not extend into deeper tissues may go into remission within a few years, while linear scleroderma lesions—especially on the head or scalp—can remain active for many years or even throughout childhood. It is important that patients who have lesions involving deeper tissues continue to be monitored at least yearly, even after treatment is stopped, because the disease can come back (relapse).

Broader Health Impacts: Associated Problems

The overall prognosis is much better for localized scleroderma than for systemic sclerosis, because life-threatening internal organ involvement is extremely rare. However, localized disease can cause disfigurement, and the skin hardening can cause discomfort and sores as well as problems such as limited joint movement. In addition, many children can have problems of other organs or tissues. Those with linear scleroderma are at a higher risk for severe growth problems, such as developing a deformed, shorter or smaller limb or portion of their face or scalp. Children with linear scleroderma lesions on their face or head can develop eye inflammation, eyelid or dental problems, headaches, seizures, and other brain problems. They need regular eye examinations and—in some cases—MRI evaluation of the brain and/or eyes. Other problems include arthritis, limited joint movement, muscle atrophy, and reflux of stomach contents. Children with pansclerotic morphea can develop chronic skin ulcers and may be at risk for squamous cell carcinoma.

Living With Illness; Lifestyle Changes

Most children with localized scleroderma don't need to make major lifestyle changes. All affected children should go to school. Some accommodations may be needed for children with severe disease affecting their ability to walk or write easily. Encourage affected children to remain active, but some activities—such as contact sports—should be limited in patients at risk for skin breakdown or in those with extremely limited movement in major joints.

Points To Remember

- Treatment for scleroderma should start as soon as possible. Treatment is more effective during the early inflammatory stage as the medicines do not directly target fibrosis.
- Children are at risk for growth problems and internal tissue involvement, so regular follow-up visits with the rheumatologist are essential to ensure that treatment is controlling inflammation and to minimize side effects from treatment.
- Children should see their pediatric rheumatologist at least once per year, because linear scleroderma can persist for many years, or come back after being inactive for several years.

Source: "Localized Scleroderma," © 2012 American College of Rheumatology.

Scleroderma (Also Known As Systemic Sclerosis)

Scleroderma is a disease affecting the skin and other organs of the body. Scleroderma is one of the autoimmune rheumatic diseases, meaning that the body's immune system is acting abnormally. The main finding in scleroderma is thickening and tightening of the skin, and inflammation and scarring of many body parts leading to problems in the lungs, kidneys, heart, intestinal system, and other areas. There is still no cure for scleroderma but effective treatments for some forms of the disease are available.

Fast Facts

- Scleroderma is relatively rare. Only 75,000 to 100,000 people in the U.S. have it. More than 75 percent of people with scleroderma are women.

- The condition affects adults and children, but it is most common in women aged 30 to 50.

- There are several types of scleroderma and related diseases and the names can be confusing. The two main types are localized (which affects the skin on the face, hands, and feet) and systemic (which can also affect blood vessels and major internal organs).

- Although the underlying cause is unknown, promising research is shedding light on the relationship between the immune system and scleroderma.

What Is Scleroderma?

Scleroderma (also known as systemic sclerosis) is a chronic disease that causes the skin to become thick and hard; a buildup of scar tissue; and damage to internal organs such as the heart and blood vessels, lungs, stomach, and kidneys. Scleroderma symptoms vary widely and they range from minor to life threatening, depending on how widespread the disease is and which parts of the body are affected.

The two main types of scleroderma are:

- **Localized scleroderma,** which usually affects only the skin, although it can spread to the muscles, joints, and bones. It does not affect other organs. In some cases, this type of scleroderma is just a cosmetic problem. Symptoms include discolored patches on the skin (a condition called morphea); or streaks or bands of thick, hard skin on the arms and legs (called linear scleroderma). When linear scleroderma occurs on the face and forehead, it is called en coup de sabre.

- **Systemic scleroderma,** which is the most serious form of the disease, affects the skin, muscles, joints, blood vessels, lungs, kidneys, heart, and other organs.

What Causes Scleroderma?

The cause of scleroderma is not known. Genetic factors (different genes) appear be important in the disease. Although exposure to certain chemicals may play a role in some people having scleroderma, the vast majority of patients with scleroderma do not have a history of exposure to any suspicious toxins. The cause of scleroderma is likely quite complicated.

Who Gets Scleroderma?

Scleroderma is relatively rare. About 75,000 to 100,000 people in the U.S. have this disease; most are women between the ages of 30 and 50. Twins and family members of those with scleroderma or other autoimmune connective tissue diseases, such as lupus, may have a slightly higher risk of getting scleroderma. Children can also develop scleroderma, but the disease is different in children than in adults.

How Is Scleroderma Diagnosed?

Diagnosis can be tricky because symptoms may be similar to those of other diseases. There is no one blood test or X-ray that can say for sure that you have scleroderma.

To make a diagnosis, a doctor will ask about your medical history, do a physical exam and possibly order lab tests and X-rays. Some symptoms he or she will look for include:

- Raynaud's phenomenon. This term refers to color changes (blue, white, and red) that occur in fingers (and sometimes toes), often after exposure to cold temperatures. It occurs when blood flow to the hands and fingers is temporarily cut off. This is one of the earliest signs of the disease; more than 90 percent of patients with scleroderma have Raynaud's. Raynaud's can lead to finger swelling, color changes, numbness, pain, skin ulcers, and gangrene on the fingers and toes.

- Skin thickening, swelling, and tightening. This is the problem that leads to the name "scleroderma" ("sclera" means hard and "derma" means skin). The skin may also become glossy or unusually dark or light in places. The disease can sometimes result in changes is personal appearance, especially in the face.

- Enlarged red blood vessels on the hands, face and around nail beds (called "telangiectasias").

- Calcium deposits in the skin or other areas.

- High blood pressure from kidney problems.

- Heartburn or other problems of the digestive tract such as difficulty swallowing food, bloating, and constipation.

- Shortness of breath.

- Joint pain.

How Is Scleroderma Treated?

While some treatments are effective in treating some aspects of this disease, there is no drug that has been clearly proven to stop, or reverse, the key symptom of skin thickening and hardening. Medications that have proven helpful in treating other autoimmune diseases, such as rheumatoid arthritis and lupus, usually don't work for people with scleroderma. Doctors aim to curb individual symptoms and prevent further complications with a combination of drugs and self-care. For example:

Raynaud's phenomenon can be treated with drugs such as calcium channel blockers, which open up narrowed blood vessels and improve circulation. To prevent further damage, it's important to keep the whole body warm, especially fingers and toes. It's also important to protect fingertips and other skin areas from injury, which can happen even during normal daily activities.

Heartburn (acid reflux) can be treated with antacid drugs, especially proton-pump inhibitors (omeprazole and others). These medications ease gastro-esophageal reflux disease (known as GERD).

Scleroderma kidney disease can be treated with blood pressure medications called "angiotensin converting enzyme inhibitors" (ACE inhibitors). These can often effectively control kidney damage if started early and use of these drugs has been a major advance for treating scleroderma.

Muscle pain and weakness can be treated with anti-inflammatory drugs such as glucocorticoids (prednisone), intravenous immunoglobulin (IVIg), and/or immunosuppressive medications. Physical therapy may be useful to maintain joint and skin flexibility.

Lung damage. There are two types of lung disease that patients with scleroderma may develop. The first type is called interstitial lung disease (scarring). There is evidence that cyclophosphamide is somewhat effective in treating the interstitial lung disease in scleroderma. Clinical trials are underway assessing the effectiveness of several other drugs for this problem.

The second type of lung disease seen in scleroderma is pulmonary arterial hypertension (high blood pressure in the arteries in the lungs). In the last 10 years, a number of drugs have become available to treat this condition, including prostacyclin-like drugs (epoprostenol, treprostinil, iloprost), the endothelin receptor antagonists (bosentan, ambrisentan), and PDE-5 inhibitors (sildenafil, vardenafil, tadalafil).

Much research is ongoing into new treatments for scleroderma. Patients and their families should know that experts remain optimistic and take comfort in the fact that work towards a cure will continue.

Broader Health Impact Of Scleroderma

Scleroderma can involve almost every organ system in the body. Although symptoms vary greatly from patient to patient, it can dramatically impact someone's life.

Patients should consult a rheumatologist—or a team of specialists—who are experienced in dealing with this complicated disease. Several other diseases that affect the skin are sometimes confused with scleroderma.

Living With Scleroderma

Living with scleroderma is quite challenging. Everyday activities can sometimes be difficult due to physical limitations and pain. Problems with digestion may require changes in diet; patients often have to eat several small meals more frequently. Patients must also keep the skin well moisturized to lessen stiffness and be careful during activities such as gardening, cooking—even opening envelopes—to avoid finger injuries. To keep the body warm, patients should dress in layers; wear socks, boots, and gloves; and avoid very cold rooms. Unfortunately, moving to a warmer climate does not necessarily lead to dramatic improvement. Exercise and/ or physical therapy may ease stiffness in the joints.

Patients must also deal with the psychological setbacks that come from living with a disease that is chronic, uncommon, and currently incurable. Because scleroderma can cause significant changes in appearance, a patient's self-esteem and self-image are almost always affected. The support of family and friends is vital in helping to maintain a good quality of life.

Points To Remember

- Scleroderma differs from person to person but can be very serious.
- There are medications, as well as steps individuals can take, to ease the symptoms of Raynaud's phenomenon, skin problems, and heartburn.
- Effective treatments are available for those with severe disease, including acute kidney disease, pulmonary hypertension, lung inflammation, and gastrointestinal problems.
- It is important to recognize and treat organ involvement early on to prevent irreversible damage.
- Patients should see physicians with specialized expertise in the care of this complex disease.
- A great deal of research is underway to find better treatments for scleroderma and, hopefully, someday a cure.

Source: "Scleroderma (Also Known As Systemic Sclerosis)," © 2012 American College of Rheumatology.

Chapter 39

Urticaria (Hives)

Hives are welts on the skin that often itch. These welts can appear on any part of the skin. Hives vary in size from as small as a pen tip to as large as a dinner plate. They may connect to form even larger welts.

A hive often goes away in 24 hours or less. New hives may appear as old ones fade, so hives may last for a few days or longer. A bout of hives usually lasts less than six weeks. These hives are called acute hives. If hives last more than six weeks, they are called chronic hives.

Acute hives often result from an allergy, but they can have many other causes.

The medical term for hives is urticaria (ur-tih-CAR-ee-uh). When large welts occur deeper under the skin, the medical term is angioedema (an-gee-oh-eh-dee-ma). This can occur with hives, and often causes the eyelids and lips to swell.

In severe cases, the throat and airway can swell, making breathing or swallowing difficult. If this occurs, the person needs emergency care right away.

Hives: Who Gets And Causes

Who gets hives?

Hives are common. Anyone can get them.

What causes hives?

An allergic reaction can trigger hives. Things that trigger commonly trigger an allergic reaction include:

- Foods: Fruits (especially citrus fruits), milk, eggs, peanuts, tree nuts, and shellfish
- Medicines
- Insect bites and stings
- Animals
- Pollen
- Touching something to which you are allergic, such as latex
- Allergy shots

Other causes of hives are:

- Infections, including colds and infections caused by some bacteria or fungi
- Some illnesses, including a type of vasculitis, lupus, and thyroid disease
- Exposure to sun (solar urticaria), heat, cold, or water
- Exercise
- Stress
- Pressure on the skin, such as from sitting too long
- Contact with chemicals
- Scratching the skin

Hives can happen within minutes of exposure to the trigger. Or you can have a delayed reaction of more than two hours.

Hives: Signs And Symptoms

The most common signs (what you see) of hives are:

- Slightly raised, pink or red swellings on the skin.
- Welts that occur alone or in a group, or connect over a large area.
- Skin swelling that subsides or goes away within 24 hours at one spot but may appear at another spot.

As for symptoms (what you feel), hives usually itch. They sometimes sting or hurt.

Some people always get hives in the same spot or spots on their body. These people often have a trigger (what causes the hives). Every time they are exposed to that trigger, they get hives.

Your dermatologist may call this type of hives fixed, which means not moving. Fixed hives may happen when a person takes a certain medicine (fixed drug eruption) or gets too much sunlight (fixed solar urticaria).

Hives: Diagnosis, Treatment, And Outcomes

How do dermatologists diagnose hives?

When a patient has hives on the skin, a dermatologist can often make the diagnosis by looking at the skin. Finding the cause of hives, however, can sometimes be hard. This is especially true for hives that have been around for more than six weeks.

To find out what is causing your hives, your dermatologist will review your health history, ask questions, and do a physical exam. You may need the following tests:

- Allergy tests (on the skin or blood tests)
- Blood work (to rule out an illness or infection)
- A skin biopsy

To perform a skin biopsy, the dermatologist removes a small piece of affected skin so that it can be examined under a microscope.

How do dermatologists treat hives?

For a mild or moderate case of hives, the most common treatment is a non-sedating (does not cause drowsiness) antihistamine. Antihistamines relieve symptoms like itching.

If you have chronic hives, your dermatologist may prescribe an antihistamine. You should take this medicine every day to prevent hives from forming. There are many antihistamines on the market. Some make you drowsy, and some do not. No one antihistamine works for everyone. Your dermatologist may combine an antihistamine with other medicines to control the hives.

Other medicines that are prescribed to treat hives include:

- Cortisones (for short-term use only because of side effects with long-term use)
- Dapsone, an antibacterial
- Other medicines that fight inflammation (redness and swelling)

Ask your dermatologist about possible side effects (health problems that can result from the medicines).

For some cases of hives or angioedema, you may need an injection of epinephrine (shot of adrenaline).

A hive often will go away in 24 hours or less, but bouts can last longer.

Outcome

A few people have chronic hives (lasting more than six weeks). Sometimes chronic hives go away on their own—often within a year. For others, hives can come and go for months or years. Children may outgrow the allergies that cause their hives.

For most people, hives are not serious. In some people, though, hives may be a sign of an internal disease. Others can get a severe swelling with hives known as angioedema. If you have hives and trouble breathing or swallowing, get emergency care right away.

Hives: Tips For Managing

When hives are mild, you may not need treatment. You can often relieve the itching by placing cool cloths on the hives, or by taking cool showers.

If you have a bad allergic reaction, like shortness of breath, talk to your doctor about a prescription medicine called an "auto-injector." This medicine stops the allergic reaction when you inject it into your thigh. Follow your doctor's advice on how to use this medicine.

Support Groups

If allergies cause your hives, you can find support groups that help people living with allergies.

Allergy Educational Support Groups

The Asthma and Allergy Foundation of America (www.aafa.org) offers support groups for young people and adults and for parents of children with allergies.

The best remedy for hives is to try to avoid whatever triggers them.

Chapter 40

Vitiligo

About Vitiligo And Its Symptoms

What is vitiligo?

Vitiligo is an autoimmune disease characterized by the loss of pigment in one or more areas of the body.

How do you pronounce the word "vitiligo"?

Vitiligo is pronounced "vittle-eye-go."

What is an autoimmune disease?

Autoimmune diseases are characterized by the body's immune system attacking its own tissue or cells—in this case, the melanocytes (pigment cells which give the skin its color). Scientists are of the opinion that in most people with autoimmune disease, the immune system is basically normal outside of the autoimmune attack. Thus, people with generalized vitiligo are thought to have otherwise healthy immune systems except for the specific immune response to melanocytes.

What is a melanocyte?

Melanocytes are the body's pigment-making cells.

About This Chapter: Information in this chapter is excerpted from "Frequently Asked Questions about Vitiligo (FAQ)," and reprinted with permission from Vitiligo Support International, © 2013. All rights reserved. For additional information, visit www.vitiligosupport.org.

What does vitiligo look like?

With vitiligo, the skin has normal texture, but the affected areas lose their pigment, resulting in irregular white spots or patches. Different types of vitiligo result in different patterns of pigment loss.

What are the symptoms of vitiligo?

The most common symptom is the loss of pigment in the skin. Less common signs include pigment loss or graying of hair on scalp, eyebrows, eyelashes, or other affected areas.

Pigment may also be lost on the tissues that line the inside of the mouth (mucous membranes) and the retina of the eye. Some of those affected by vitiligo experience intense itching at the site of depigmentation during active stages.

What are the different types of vitiligo?

Segmental Vitiligo (SV) most often begins at an early age and affects only one area, on one side of the body, such as one side of the mouth or neck. It generally spreads fairly quickly at the onset, then slows and remains stable after a year or so. More than half of those affected by SV will also have patches of white hair.

Non-Segmental Vitiligo (NSV) includes all types of vitiligo except segmental, such as focal vitiligo (pigment loss limited to one, or very few areas), acrofacial vitiligo (pigment loss occurring only on the face and extremities such as hands and feet), and the most common, generalized vitiligo (pigment loss on both side of the body in a mirror-like image, such as both hands or both knees). NSV typically begins on areas such as the hands, wrists, around the eyes or mouth, or on the feet, then spreads to areas such as the neck, chest, knees and legs. NSV is considered to be progressive, but has cycles of spreading and cycles of stability. Also, while it is uncommon, a person with SV can later develop NSV.

Mixed Vitiligo (MV) begins as segmental vitiligo, then later progresses into non-segmental vitiligo, becoming "mixed vitiligo."

Will the vitiligo patches spread over time? Will they get larger?

Generalized vitiligo is a progressive disease resulting in somewhat unpredictable cycles of spreading and cycles of stability throughout life. For some, it begins slowly with only a few areas of the body affected; for others, it begins rapidly, with many areas affected by both large and small patches of pigment loss. Many patients report going many years without new patches developing, then experience pigment loss years later. Others report spontaneous repigmentation, with no treatment at all.

Who is affected by vitiligo?

Vitiligo affects about .05 percent to 1 percent of the world population, including both genders and all races. Vitiligo can start at any age, but about half of those with vitiligo develop it before the age of 20, and about 95 percent before age 40. Approximately 20 percent of vitiligo patients have a family member with the same condition. However, only 5 percent to 7 percent of children with a parent who has vitiligo will develop it.

Is vitiligo at all contagious?

Vitiligo is NOT contagious. It is a genetic disease, caused by inheritance of multiple causal genes simultaneously, possibly in different combinations in different people, plus exposure to environmental risk factors or triggers that are not yet known.

Cause And Effect

What causes vitiligo?

The likelihood of developing vitiligo results from different combinations of susceptibility genes, even in the same family. Different family members inherit different genetic combinations, just as they do for height or intelligence. Even among identical twins, both develop vitiligo only one-fourth of the time. Identical twins share all their genes in common, but they don't share their environmental exposures and other life-events. While it is known that environmental triggers are involved, it is still uncertain as to what they are, with stress (physical and emotional), skin trauma, and exposure to certain chemicals being possible triggers.

Doctors And Treatments

How is vitiligo diagnosed?

The doctor usually begins by asking the person about his or her medical history. Important factors are a family history of vitiligo or other autoimmune diseases; a rash, sunburn, or other skin trauma at the site of vitiligo two to three months before depigmentation started; stress or physical illness. The doctor may take a small sample (biopsy) of the affected skin, and/or a blood sample to do lab work that checks for thyroid antibodies/disease, lupus, vitamin D levels, and other conditions that may affect general health or autoimmune status. The doctor may also use a Woods light (specialized black light) to confirm vitiligo, as vitiligo will glow under this light.

I was told vitiligo could not be treated. Is that correct?

No, that is incorrect. While no treatment currently available works for everyone, there are a variety of treatments that work for many affected by vitiligo.

What treatment options are available?

The treatments for vitiligo include a variety of topicals, light therapies, systemic steroids, surgery, and de-pigmentation techniques. Traditional therapies include Psoralen + Ultraviolet A Light (PUVA), and steroids. Modern therapies include Narrow Band-Ultraviolet B Light (NB-UVB), topical immunomodulators (tacrolimus, pimecrolimus), analogues of vitamin D3, excimer laser, and surgery/transplantation.

How long does it take to treat vitiligo? When should I expect results?

Treatment results will vary by person and type of vitiligo. Some people will begin to see results within three to six months. Others may not see results for eight months. The rule of thumb is that you will need to allow at least three to six months before you begin to see results from ANY treatment. Additionally, you should expect to treat for up to two years or longer in order to see good results. It is vital to use any treatment consistently and correctly. If you don't use a treatment as directed by your physician, it can take much longer to work or it may not work at all.

What is PUVA?

PUVA stands for **P**soralen plus **U**ltra**V**iolet **A** light, and is a form of phototherapy using long wave UVA light in combination with either a photosensitizing pill or a topical solution known as a psoralen. When using the pill form, the psoralen sensitizes the skin and eyes for up to 24 hours. To prevent the risk of cataracts, patients must wear approved wraparound sunglasses, indoors and out, for up to 24 hours after taking the tablets. PUVA is generally considered a less effective therapy, with more side effects, than NB-UVB.

What is PUVA-SOL?

For patients who cannot go to a facility with a UVA lightbox, the doctor may prescribe psoralen to be used with natural sunlight exposure. The doctor will give the patient careful instructions on carrying out treatment at home and monitor the patient during scheduled checkups.

What is narrowband UVB? (NB-UVB)

NB-UVB, now considered the gold standard of treatment for vitiligo covering more than 20 percent of the body, is a more recent vitiligo treatment than PUVA, and uses the portion of the UVB spectrum from 311-313 nanometers (nm). This light spectrum has been determined to help stimulate pigment cells to produce melanocytes in less time than it takes to burn the skin. NB-UVB is sometimes used in combination with other topical treatments, but is effective for many on its own. NB-UVB can be used on children old enough to stand still and keep goggles on.

What is an excimer laser?

The excimer laser is a targeted NB machine typically using the 308 nm portion of the spectrum. Laser can be very effective for smaller areas of stable vitiligo. As it treats a small area, it is inefficient for larger areas or percentages. Results from laser treatments frequently occur more quickly than with other treatments. Because laser treatments are expensive, it is typically only used on stable vitiligo because when the vitiligo is active there is a greater chance of pigment being lost afterwards. Hands and feet are often not treated with laser because it is less effective there. Treatments are generally two to three times per week.

How are topical steroids used for vitiligo?

Generally, use of topical steroids in widespread vitiligo is considered impractical because of the greater risk of associated adverse side effects due to the significant amount of skin that would be treated. However, research has shown that very potent or potent (class 1 and class 2) topical corticosteroids can be used either intermittently or on a short-term basis to re-pigment vitiligo-affected skin in adults. Most physicians prescribe less potent topical steroids for use by children.

What are Protopic and Elidel?

Protopic (tacrolimus), and Elidel (pimecrolimus) are both classified as immunomodulators, and are prescribed in their topical form for vitiligo. An immunomodulator is not the same as a steroid; it works by modulating (reducing) the immune response (where applied), allowing the melanocytes to once again grow and flourish.

What is V-Tar?

V- Tar is a prescription coal tar product used for treating vitiligo. V-Tar is applied once weekly and is one of the few treatments for vitiligo that does not need some form of light therapy to work. However, because of its photo-sensitizing properties, patients using V-tar are advised to avoid direct sunlight, or use a sunscreen, on the treated areas for three days post application. It is only available from the one compounding pharmacy that developed it.

What is surgical therapy for vitiligo?

Repigmentation surgery has the goal of transplanting functional melanocytes (pigment cells) to the depigmented area. This transplantation can be done through one of several methods, each of which harvests the melanocytes in a different way.

When is surgical therapy an option?

Although medical therapy has improved considerably in the last years, some people fail to sufficiently re-pigment through medical treatment. Surgical therapy can provide higher re-pigmentation rates for difficult-to-treat localized areas in selected patients, and can be used to treat generalized disease as well. Those considered the best candidates and most likely to experience a high rate of repigmentation from surgical therapies are those with stable, segmental, or localized vitiligo.

What types of surgical therapies are available?

There are two types of surgical transplantation (grafts) available:

1. Tissue Grafts
2. Cellular Grafts

With tissue grafts, only a limited surface area can be treated, but with good results in the majority of cases. Grafting is suitable for stable patches and can be done in multiple ways using mini-punch grafts, thin-split thickness grafts, and suction blister grafting.

There are two methods of cellular grafting:

- Cultured
- Non-cultured

Cultured cellular grafts involve the doctor taking a sample of normal pigmented skin and placing it in a laboratory dish containing a special cell-culture solution to grow melanocytes. When the melanocytes in the culture solution have multiplied, the doctor transplants them to the depigmented skin patches. These in vitro (in the lab) culture techniques can be used to treat extensive areas of depigmented skin as well as localized areas. Extremities of peripheral body areas, such as the dorsal (tops of the) fingers, ankles, forehead, and hairline, and bony prominences do not respond well.

Non-cultured grafts are performed all in one surgery and always include both melanocytes and keratinocytes. The Henry Ford Hospital (HFH) in Detroit now performs this procedure.

HFH reports that this method can cover an area 10 times the size of the donor sample taken. This method also requires less equipment and is an easier process, making it likely that it will be more readily available at some point.

There are two cellular transplantation techniques:

- Transplantation of melanocytes and keratinocytes
- Transplantation of melanocytes only

Transplantation of melanocytes and keratinocytes (non-cultured or cultured procedure): The initial step in this procedure is harvesting a small donor skin sample to provide cells for an epidermal or melanocytes/keratinocytes suspension.

For a non-cultured transplant, the suspension is then placed over the abraded area on the recipient site. The advantage of this method is the relative simplicity, but cost can still be a factor. Reported side effects include spotty pigmentation or failure to repigment. Scarring, infection, or poor wound healing have also been reported.

Cultured transplantation of melanocytes and keratinocytes requires the cell suspension be seeded in culture flasks with an appropriate culture media. Thin epidermal sheets are obtained three weeks later, which are removed from the culture vessel and transferred to the recipient site previously denuded by one of various procedures.

Transplantation of melanocytes only is always a cultured procedure and follows the same guidelines as the cultured method above.

What is depigmentation?

While some people totally depigment through the natural progression of their vitiligo, others make the choice to depigment. If a patient would like to consider this option, their doctor may request they begin with a psychological screening to determine that this decision is one they fully understand and are emotionally prepared for. It is generally only used in cases of advanced vitiligo, where there is more than 50 percent loss of pigment, though some physicians may allow its use with a lower percentage when a great deal of the vitiligo is located in the more visible areas.

If their doctor determines they are a candidate for this treatment, they begin the fairly simple process by using a topical prescription called monobenzyl ether of hydroquinone (MBEH). It is important to understand that this is a systemic treatment, meaning that once the cream is applied to the skin, it will cause depigmentation in remote areas away from the site of application.

This prescription is a compounded cream for use only by those with extensive vitiligo and is available in strengths of 10%, 20% (most often) or 30% or 40%. This cream has been around for at least 30 years, and was formerly manufactured with the trade name of "Benoquin," but is now most commonly known by its generic name "monobenzone."

The patient will apply the cream twice daily, perhaps increasing the strength of the active ingredients and/or the coverage area, over a period of a year or more, until the normally pigmented skin has faded to match the vitiligo spots, creating an overall pale appearance. The paleness is not a stark white, as many fear, but rather a slightly pink tone.

Is it safe to use all treatments on the face and around the eyes?

Research has shown that NB-UVB eyelid phototherapy is a safe and effective treatment and does not penetrate the eyelid. For their patients old enough to understand the importance of keeping the eyes closed, many doctors permit removing the goggles for part of the time to expose depigmented areas around the eyes. Care must be taken however, not to over expose the eyelid, as the very thin skin will not tolerate a high exposure time. Eye protection is always required when using any type of psoralen and/or UVA light, such as with PUVA therapy.

Most topical treatments prescribed for vitiligo can be used on the face; however, care must be taken to prevent them from getting into the eye. Due to their many potential side effects, potent topical steroids are generally not prescribed for use on the face, except for very short periods of time while under careful supervision of the prescribing physician. Monobenzone for depigmentation is generally not used on the face due to the potential for a rash forming.

Cosmetics And Other Products

Many people with vitiligo feel more confident in public when they cover their vitiligo with some type of camouflage or makeup. There are much better corrective cosmetics on the market today than in the past that work well for men as well as women. Some choose to cover their vitiligo every day, others just for special occasions.

What type of cosmetics are available to cover vitiligo spots?

Cosmetic options for vitiligo include corrective cosmetic creams; homemade stain made from food coloring and rubbing alcohol; DHA (dihydroxyacetone)-based sunless tanners available in cream, spray, or airbrush (home or salon); and non-DHA, custom color products (airbrush or stipple).

Emotional, Social, And Relationship Issues

The change in appearance caused by vitiligo can affect a person's emotional and psychological well-being and may cause an alteration in their lifestyle, becoming less active in social activities. Many people find that the emotional stress increases as vitiligo develops on visible areas of the body such as the face, hands, arms, feet, or on the genitals. It is not uncommon for those with vitiligo to feel embarrassed, ashamed, depressed, or worried about how others will react. Adolescents, who are already concerned about their appearance, can be devastated. Patients need to let their doctor know if they are feeling depressed because doctors and other mental health professionals can help with the depression.

One of the first steps in coping is finding a doctor who is knowledgeable about vitiligo and current treatments, and is capable of providing emotional support. Patients should also learn as much as possible about vitiligo and treatment choices so that they can participate in making important decisions about their medical care. This proactive approach will help them regain control of their life rather than allowing vitiligo to make the rules. It's also important to establish support with family and friends and to talk with others who have vitiligo. Organizations like Vitiligo Support International can help.

Part Five
Skin Injuries

Chapter 41

Scrapes, Cuts, And Bruises

Cuts, Scratches, And Scrapes

You wipe out on your skateboard. The knife you're using slices your finger instead of the tomato. Your new puppy doesn't know how sharp his baby teeth are.

You might think a cut or scrape is no big deal, but any time the skin gets broken, there's a risk of infection. So it helps to understand how to care for cuts and scrapes at home—and know when you need to see a doctor.

What To Do

Many small cuts, scrapes, or abrasions will heal well without medical care. Here's what to do if the injury isn't serious:

- **Stop bleeding by pressing a clean, soft cloth against the wound for a few minutes.** If the wound is bleeding a lot, you'll need to hold pressure for longer (sometimes up to 15 minutes). If the wound is small, the bleeding should stop in a few minutes as the blood's clotting factors do their work to seal the wound.

- **As you keep the pressure on and the wound, avoid the urge to peek.** Lifting the bandage may start the bleeding again.

About This Chapter: "Cuts, Scratches, And Scrapes," November 2011, and "Bruises," May 2009, reprinted with permission from www.kidshealth.org. This information was provided by KidsHealth®, one of the largest resources online for medically reviewed health information written for parents, kids, and teens. For more articles like this, visit www.KidsHealth.org, or www.TeensHealth.org. Copyright © 1995-2012 The Nemours Foundation. All rights reserved.

Top Things To Know About Cuts And Scrapes

- See a doctor if a cut doesn't stop bleeding, if it is wide or deep or doesn't look like it's going to close on it's own, or if you're bitten by an animal or another person.

- If you can't get all the dirt out of a cut or scrape, call your doctor. Even if the cut or scrape is small or minor, dirt can cause infection.

- Keep cuts clean, dry, and covered. Watch for signs of infection. If you think a wound is infected, call a doctor.

- **Clean the wound.** Run warm water over the cut for five minutes. Then use soap to gently wash the skin around the cut or scrape thoroughly. If there's dirt or debris in the wound (like gravel from a scrape), remove it if you can—a soft, damp cloth can help. Cleaning the wound helps get infection-causing bacteria out of the injured area. *If you can't get all the dirt out, call your doctor's office.*

- **If you want, put a light layer of an antibiotic ointment around the cut to kill germs.** Make sure you're not allergic to the medications in the ointment.

- **Dry the area lightly and cover it with gauze or other type of bandage.** A bandage helps prevent germs. If the bandage gets wet or dirty, change it right away.

- **Each day, take off the bandage and gently wash the injury.** Watch for signs of infection.

- **To prevent infection and reduce scarring, don't pick at the scab or skin around the wound.**

When To Get Help

If blood is spurting out of a cut or it won't stop bleeding, get a parent or call your doctor right away. Cover the wound with a sterile bandage or clean cloth. If the blood soaks through, don't remove the first bandage—put a new covering on top of it. Raising the injured body part above your head (or holding it up as high as you can) may help slow the bleeding.

If a wound is very long or deep, or if its edges are far apart, a doctor will need to close it with stitches. A doctor or nurse will numb your skin with an anesthetic shot (sometimes they put an anesthetic cream on the skin first to numb the area). If you hate the idea of a shot, it can help to keep in mind that getting multiple stitches feels like getting multiple shots, so you're better off feeling only one!

If you get stitches, you'll probably need to go back to the doctor in 5 to 10 days to get them taken out (some stitches dissolve on their own). To remove stitches, a doctor or nurse will snip the thread with scissors and gently pull out the threads. It feels ticklish and a little funny, but usually doesn't hurt.

Doctors sometimes close small, straight cuts on certain parts of the body with medical glue or Steri-Strips (thin pieces of tape). Glue and Steri-Strips will dissolve or fall off on their own.

Getting a cut usually means that there will be some scarring. If your cut needs to be stitched or glued but you don't see a doctor in time, your scar may be more noticeable.

Avoiding Infection

Let a parent, coach, or other adult know if you get injured. You'll especially want to tell someone if you cut yourself on something dirty or rusty, if you are bleeding, or if you get bitten or scratched (by an animal or a person!).

Bites that break the skin need medical care. Germs from animal or human saliva can get into the wound, and you will usually need antibiotics to prevent infection. Your doctor or nurse will also want to make sure the animal didn't have rabies.

Certain cuts or bites could lead to a tetanus infection if your tetanus shots are not up to date. You (or your mom or dad) will need to check your medical records to be sure that you have had a tetanus shot recently. If you haven't, you will probably need to get one when the cut is repaired.

Signs Of Infection

Sometimes, a cut, scratch, or scrape starts out as no big deal, but then gets infected. A skin infection happens when there are too many germs for your body's white blood cells to handle.

If you notice any of these signs of infection, call your doctor right away:

- Expanding redness around the wound
- Yellow or greenish-colored pus or cloudy wound drainage
- Red streaking spreading from the wound
- Increased swelling, tenderness, or pain around the wound
- Fever

The doctor will prescribe antibiotics to help your body fight off the infection.

Most of the time small cuts, scratches, and abrasions go away on their own, thanks to your body's amazing ability to heal itself. If a cut looks serious or infected, though, see a doctor.

Bruises

Man, does that hurt! You took that hill too quickly on your bike, lost your balance on your blades, or someone on the other soccer team missed the ball completely and kicked you right in the shin. The pain is bad enough, but the bruise left behind is pretty ugly. It's nothing new; you've had a bruise or two before. But what exactly is a bruise?

What Is A Bruise?

A bruise, also called a **contusion** (pronounced: kun-**too**-zhen) or an **ecchymosis** (pronounced: eh-ky-**moe**-sis), happens when a part of the body is struck and the muscle fibers and connective tissue underneath are crushed but the skin doesn't break. When this occurs, blood from the ruptured **capillaries** (small blood vessels) near the skin's surface escapes by leaking out under the skin. With no place to go, the blood gets trapped, forming a red or purplish mark that's tender when you touch it—a bruise.

Bruises can happen for many reasons, but most are the result of bumping and banging into things—or having things bump and bang into you. Fortunately, as anyone who's ever sported a shiner knows, the mark isn't permanent.

How Long Do Bruises Last?

You know how a bruise changes color over time? That's your body fixing the bruise by breaking down and reabsorbing the blood, which causes the bruise to go through many colors of the rainbow before it eventually disappears. You can pretty much guess the age of a bruise just by looking at its color:

- When you first get a bruise, it's kind of reddish as the blood appears under the skin.
- Within one or two days, the hemoglobin (an iron-containing substance that carries oxygen) in the blood changes and your bruise turns bluish-purple or even blackish.
- After 5 to 10 days, the bruise turns greenish or yellowish.
- Then, after 10 or 14 days, it turns yellowish-brown or light brown.

Finally, after about two weeks, your bruise fades away.

Who Gets Bruises?

Anyone can get a bruise. Some people bruise easily, whereas others don't. Why? Bruising depends on several things, such as:

- How tough the skin tissue is

- Whether someone has certain diseases or conditions

- Whether a person's taking certain medications

Also, blood vessels tend to become fragile as people get older, which is why elderly people tend to bruise more easily.

What Can I Do To Help Myself Feel Better?

It's hard to prevent bruises, but you can help speed the healing process. When you get a bruise, you can use stuff you find right in your freezer to help the bruise go away faster. Applying cold when you first get a bruise helps reduce its size by slowing down the blood that's flowing to the area, which decreases the amount of blood that ends up leaking into the tissues. It also keeps the inflammation and swelling down. All you have to do is apply cold to the bruise for half an hour to an hour at a time for a day or two after the bruise appears.

You don't need to buy a special cold pack, although they're great to keep on hand in the freezer. Just get some ice, put it in a plastic bag, and wrap the bag in a cloth or a towel and place it on the bruise (it isn't such a good idea to apply the ice directly to the skin).

Another trick is to use a bag of frozen vegetables. It doesn't matter what kind—carrots, peas, lima beans, whatever—as long as they're frozen. A bag of frozen vegetables is easy to apply to the bruise because it can form to the shape of the injured area. Also, like a cold pack, it can be used and refrozen again and again (just pick your least-favorite vegetables as it's not a good idea to keep thawing and freezing veggies that you plan to eat!).

Another way to help heal your bruise is to elevate the bruised area above the level of your heart. In other words, if the bruise is on your shin, lie down on a couch or bed and prop up your leg. This will slow the flow of the red blood cells to the bruise because more of the blood in your leg will flow back toward the rest of your body instead of leaking out into the tissues of your leg. If you keep standing, more blood will flow to your bruised shin and the bruise will grow faster.

When To See A Doctor

Minor bruises are easily treated, but it's probably best to talk to a doctor if:

- A bruise doesn't go away after two weeks.

- You bruise often and you haven't been bumping into things.

- Bruises seem to develop for no known reasons.

- A bruise is getting more painful.

- Your bruise is swelling.

- You can't move a joint.

- The bruise is near your eye.

Can Bruises Be Prevented?

Bruises are kind of hard to avoid completely, but if you're playing sports, riding your bike, inline skating, or doing anything where you might bump, bang, crash, or smash into something—or something might bump, bang, crash, or smash into you—it's smart to wear protective gear like pads, shin guards, and helmets. Taking just a few extra seconds to put on that gear might save you from a couple of weeks of aches and pains (not to mention save your life if the accident's really serious)!

Chapter 42

Stitches

How Should I Care For My Stitches (Sutures)?

If you have stitches (sutures), make sure that you:

- Keep them clean and dry.
- Keep an eye on the wound (where the stitches are) for any increase in redness, swelling, or pain.

This will reduce your risk of developing an infection.

Your health professional should tell you how to care for your wound. If you are unsure what to do, ask your healthcare team for advice.

Protect Your Stitches

It's important not to scratch your stitches as, even though they are strong, you scratching may damage them.

If you have stitches, avoid contact sports like football or hockey, to give your wound the best possible chance to heal.

You should also not go swimming until your wound has healed and your stitches have been removed.

About This Chapter: "How should I care for my stitches (sutures)?" and "How long will my stitches (sutures) take to dissolve?" reprinted from NHS Choices, www.nhs.uk. Reproduced by kind permission of the Department of Health, © 2013.

If your child has stitches, don't let them play with water, mud, sand, and paint. Playing with things like this could cause the wound area to get dirty or sore or cause an infection. Children may also be advised to avoid PE (gym class) at school until their wound has healed.

Signs Of infection

As well as protecting your stitches, watch out for any signs of infection such as:

- Swelling

- Increased redness around the wound

- Pus or bleeding from the wound

- The wound feeling warm

- An unpleasant smell from the wound

- Increasing pain

- A high temperature (fever)

If you have any of the symptoms above, speak to your family doctor.

Removing Stitches

You will be told if you need to return to your family doctor or a nurse to have your stitches removed. For example:

- Stitches on your head: You'll need to return after 3 to 5 days.

- Stitches over joints, such as your knees or elbows: You'll need to return after 10 to 14 days.

- Stitches on other parts of your body: You'll need to return after 7 to 10 days.

Some stitches are made of dissolvable (absorbable) material and will disappear on their own.

How Long Will My Stitches (Sutures) Take To Dissolve?

It depends on what they're made from. Most dissolvable stitches start to break down within one to two weeks. However, it could take several months before your stitches disappear completely. After the wound has healed, it may be possible for a nurse to remove the loose ends of the dissolvable stitches, to speed up the process.

Ask your surgeon or the healthcare professional treating you if they can tell you:

- What kind of stitches you've been given
- How long they will take to dissolve

What Are Dissolvable Stitches?

Stitches are classed as dissolvable or absorbable if they lose most of their strength within 60 days. The stitches are dissolved by:

- Enzymes in your body tissues (enzymes are proteins that speed up and control chemical reactions in your body)
- Hydrolysis (a chemical reaction with the water inside your body)

What Are Dissolvable Stitches Made Of?

In the U.K., most dissolvable stitches are made of:

- Polyglactin: This should lose 25 percent of its strength after two weeks, 50 percent of its strength after three weeks, and fully dissolve after three months.
- Polyglycolic acid: This should lose 40 percent of its strength after one week, 95 percent of its strength after four weeks, and fully dissolve after three to four months.

There are several other different types of stitches. In general, if your stitches are dissolvable, they should start to break down within four weeks. Some may take six months to disappear completely.

When Are Dissolvable Stitches Used?

Dissolvable stitches may be used on deep surgical wounds or surface wounds. They are normally used for deep wounds, below the surface of your skin. For example, they may be used during heart surgery or a transplant operation.

Dissolvable stitches are also used for wounds on the skin's surface. For example, they may be used after childbirth, to repair tears in the perineum (the skin between the vagina and anus).

One study found that when used to repair perineum tears, polyglactin stitches disappeared within three months and polyglycolic acid stitches disappeared within four months.

Dissolvable stitches will keep the wound closed until it's fully healed, and will then slowly disappear.

If they are still bothering you after the wound has healed, make an appointment with a nurse at your local clinic. They will be able to gently remove any loose ends that are visible.

What Else Can Be Used To Close A Wound?

Other methods of keeping a wound closed include:

- Stitches that don't dissolve

- Clips

- Staples

These will need to be removed by a healthcare professional when the wound has begun to heal.

Chapter 43

Scars

The skin is a seamless organ protecting our body from infection. Throughout our lives, we have experiences that injure our skin, leaving behind a scar. Scars depend on many factors. These include: the depth and size of the wound, your age, genetic factors, and even your sex and ethnicity. There are four main types of scars and various treatments can help reduce their size and appearance. Before you begin, however, remember this basic truth: Scars will never completely disappear.

What are the four main types of scars?

1. **Hypertrophic Scars:** These are raised, red scars that are similar to keloids (see below), but do not extend beyond the original injury site. Possible treatments include steroid injections and laser surgery.

2. **Keloids:** These scars protrude from the skin and extend beyond the original injury site and are due to overproduction of certain cells. Over time, keloids may affect mobility. Possible treatments include surgical scar removal, laser surgery or steroid injections. Smaller keloids can be removed with cryotherapy (freezing therapy using liquid nitrogen). You can also prevent keloid formation by using pressure treatment, silicone gel. Keloids are more common in darker skin types, specifically people of African or Asian descent.

3. **Contracture Scars:** These scars cause tightening of skin that can impair the ability to move. These can happen after a burn. Additionally, this type of scar may go deeper to affect muscles and nerves.

About This Chapter: "Scars," © 2012 The Cleveland Clinic Foundation, 9500 Euclid Avenue, Cleveland, OH 44195. All rights reserved. Reprinted with permission. Additional information is available from the Cleveland Clinic Health Information Center, 216-444-3771, toll-free 800-223-2273 extension 43771, or at http://my.clevelandclinic.org/health.

4. **Acne Scars:** Any type of acne can leave behind scars. There are many types of acne scars, ranging from deep pits to scars that are angular or wavelike in appearance. Treatment depends on the type of scars.

What are possible treatments?

Over-The-Counter Or Prescription Creams, Ointments, Or Gels: These products may reduce scars that are caused from surgical incisions, other injuries, or wounds. If you are under the care of a dermatologist or plastic surgeon, ask your physician for recommendations. Treatment options include corticosteroids or antihistamine creams if your scars cause itching and are sensitive. Likewise, if you have scarring as a result of acne, you should ask your dermatologist for specific recommendations for treatment of the acne and type of scarring. Your doctor may also recommend intralesional steroid injections, pressure dressings, or silicone gel sheeting to prevent acne scars and to help treat existing scars.

Surgical Scar Removal: There are many options under this category, depending on your particular case, including skin grafts, excision, or laser surgery. When looking into surgery, discuss with your doctor whether you will have local anesthesia with an oral sedative or general anesthesia. If you've recently undergone plastic, cosmetic, or other surgery that has caused your scars, it is best that you wait at least one year before making a decision about scar removal treatment. Many scars fade and become less noticeable over time.

Injections: In the case of protruding scars such as keloids or hypertrophic scars, your doctor may elect to use steroid injections to flatten the scars. Such injections can be used as a stand-alone treatment or in conjunction with other treatments.

Laser Surgery: Vascular (blood vessel) specific lasers may be used to lighten flat or raised scars that are pink to purple in color. Vascular laser treatment may also facilitate the flattening of raised scars.

Will insurance cover scar removal treatments?

If your scar is impairing you physically, your insurance plan may cover the cost. You can ask your doctor to write a letter detailing your particular case. He or she can also take photos to support your case. If you are undergoing scar removal treatment for cosmetic purposes, you will likely have to pay for it yourself. If your scars resulted from cosmetic surgery, your insurance company may or may not pay for treatment. Some plans will not cover treatments that arise from elective surgery that is not medically necessary. It is best to check with your insurance plan.

Chapter 44

Scar Removal

Different Types Of Acne

Scars from acne can seem like double punishment—first you had to deal with the pimples, now you have marks as a reminder.

It helps to understand the different kinds of acne so you can figure out what to do about different types of scarring: Acne lesions or pimples happen when the hair follicles (or "pores") on the skin become plugged with oil and dead skin cells. A plugged follicle is the perfect place for bacteria to grow and create the red bumps and pus-filled red bumps known as pimples.

Acne comes in different forms:

- Mild acne, which refers to the whiteheads or blackheads that most of us get at various times
- Moderately severe acne, which includes red inflamed pimples called **papules** and red pimples with white centers called **pustules**
- Severe acne, which causes **nodules**—painful, pus-filled cysts or lumps—to appear under the skin

Most serious scarring is caused by the more severe forms of acne, with nodules more likely to leave permanent scars than other types of acne.

The best approach is to get treatment for acne soon after it appears to prevent further severe acne and more scarring. If you have nodules, see your doctor or dermatologist for treatment.

Treating Acne Scars

Most of the time, those reddish or brownish acne marks that are left behind after a pimple eventually fade with no need for treatment. Picking or squeezing acne can increase the risk for scarring, though.

Acne scars take two forms:

1. Scars with a gradual dip or depression (sometimes called "rolling" scars)

2. Scars that are deep and narrow

A person's acne needs to be under control before scars can be treated.

Mild Vs. Severe Scarring

Treatments depend on how severe the scars are. In some cases, a doctor or dermatologist may suggest a **chemical peel** or **microdermabrasion** to help improve the appearance of scarred areas. These milder treatments can be done right in the office.

If you have serious scarring from previous bouts with acne, there are several things you can do:

- **Laser Resurfacing:** This procedure can be done in the doctor's or dermatologist's office. The laser removes the damaged top layer of skin and tightens the middle layer, leaving skin smoother. It can take anywhere from a few minutes to an hour. The doctor will try to lessen any pain by first numbing the skin with local anesthesia. It usually takes between 3 and 10 days for the skin to heal completely.

- **Dermabrasion:** This treatment uses a rotating wire brush or spinning diamond instrument to wear down the surface of the skin. As the skin heals, a new, smoother layer replaces the abraded skin. It may take a bit longer for skin to heal using dermabrasion— usually between 10 days and 3 weeks.

- **Fractional Laser Therapy:** This type of treatment works at a deeper level than laser resurfacing or dermabrasion, Because fractional laser therapy doesn't wound the top layer of tissue, healing time is shorter. Someone who has had this type of treatment may just look a bit sunburned for a couple of days.

For "rolling" scars, doctors sometimes inject material under the scar to raise it to the level of normal skin. Finally, in some cases, a doctor may recommend surgery to remove deeply indented scars.

One thing you shouldn't do to deal with acne scars is load up your face with masks or fancy lotions—these won't help and may irritate your skin further, making the scars red and even more noticeable.

If you have a red or brownish mark on your face that you got from a bad zit, it should eventually fade. However, it may take 12 months or longer. Talk to your doctor if you're upset about acne marks; he or she may have advice on what you can do.

Chapter 45

Burn Injuries

Types Of Burn Injuries

- **Thermal Burns:** Can be caused by flame, heat, or contact with a hot object.

- **Chemical Burns:** These burns most often occur in industrial settings; however, they can also be caused by common household cleaners and swimming pool chemicals. Many times, chemical burns do not appear serious at first, but become worse as they continue to react with the exposed tissue.

- **Scald Burns:** Scalds are produced by hot liquids such as water or cooking oil. These are the most common burns seen in children. Elderly persons are also at risk especially when their sensitivity to heat or cold is diminished.

- **Electrical Burns:** In addition to the actual burn, electricity can cause serious internal injuries that are not immediately visible to emergency personnel or other healthcare providers. Electrical burns can cause everything from heart attack and neurological damage to broken bones and ruptured eardrums. Electrical current can cause either a flash of flame or electrocution. Electrocution injuries are always much worse than they appear. With electrocution, even a small dime-sized burn can place a person at risk for losing a limb.

Classification Of Burn Injuries

First-Degree Burn

This is also called a superficial burn injury. It looks like a typical sunburn injury: a bit pink, a bit sore and may make the victim feel a bit dehydrated. Only the very outer layer of skin (epidermis) has been damaged. The deeper skin structures are still intact. There are no open wounds. Sunburn

---

Young Worker Safety In Restaurants

Burns: Potential Hazard

Remember: Child labor laws do not permit workers younger than 16 to cook, except at soda fountains, lunch counters, snack bars, and cafeteria serving counters.

Burn injuries are common among teen employees in restaurants. Young workers who work as fry cooks are at special risk for burn injuries. Factors such as inexperience and the pressure to keep up during busy periods can lead to potential accidents. Other hazards include exposure to:

- Hot oil, grease, and steam from hot surfaces, hot food and beverages, and equipment such as stoves, grills, steamers, and fryers. Deep fat fryers are the number one cause of burns.

Young Worker Solutions

Employers have the primary responsibility for protecting the safety and health of their workers. Employees are responsible for following the safe work practices of their employers.

Follow all safety procedures and wear all protective equipment provided by your employer and be trained in the proper use of equipment, for example:

- Do wear long-sleeved cotton shirts and pants when cooking. A clean, dry, properly worn apron or uniform can protect you from burns and hot oil splashes.
- Do not cook without wearing protective clothing, even in hot temperatures or environments.
- Use appropriate hand protection when hands are exposed to hazards such as cuts, lacerations, and thermal burns. Use oven mitts or potholders when handling hot items, and steel mesh or Kevlar gloves when cutting.
- Learn to use equipment and personal protective equipment properly and safely. For example, if cooking with steamers and pasta boilers:
  - **Use** tongs and oven mitts to remove hot items from steamers or pasta boilers.
  - **Place** hot steamed items on trays to carry, rather than carrying steamed containers across the floor, leaving a trail of dripping hot water that may cause slips and falls.

or tanning beds are usually the cause of a first-degree burn. First-degree burns usually heal in a few days. Medical care is usually not required unless it involves most of the body and you're dehydrated, or are having problems with pain control. Consult your doctor if you're concerned.

When someone suffers a first-degree burn they should:

- Drink plenty of fluids

- Apply lotion to dry skin areas as they are healing

- **Open** ovens or steamers by standing to the side, keeping the door between you and the open steamer.
- **Open** the top steamer first when steamers are stacked, and then the lower one to prevent being burned from the rising steam.
- **Do not** stand above steaming items or equipment. Steam can burn. Do not reach above an oven or steamer. Hot air and steam rises and you could be burned.
- **Do not** open cookers and steam ovens when they are under pressure.

- Check hot foods on stoves or in the microwave carefully. Uncover a container of steaming materials by lifting the lid open away from your face.
- Place sealed cooking pouches in boiling water carefully to avoid splashing.
- Assume that pots, pot handles, and utensils in pots are hot and use oven mitts when handling them. Use long gloves for deep ovens.
- Adjust burner flames to cover only the bottom of the pan. Avoid overcrowding on range tops.
- Wear sturdy footwear that is slip resistant and not canvas or open-toed to protect the feet in case hot liquids are spilled on shoes.
- Ask for help when moving or carrying a heavy pot of hot liquid off the burner.
- Do not allow pot handles or cooking utensils to stick out from counters or stove fronts. Keep pot handles away from burners.
- Avoid overfilling pots and pans.
- Do not clean vents over grill areas if the grill is hot. Clean vents the next morning before turning on for the day.
- Do not use metal containers, foil, or utensils in a microwave oven.
- Do not pour or spill water or ice into oil, especially hot oil. It will cause splattering.
- Do not leave hot oil or grease unattended.
- Do not use a wet cloth to lift lids from hot pots.
- Do not lean over pots of boiling liquid.

Source: Excerpted from "Young Worker Safety In Restaurants," Occupational Safety and Health Administration, U.S. Department of Labor, available at http://www.osha.gov/SLTC/youth/restaurant/cooking.html, accessed February 22, 2013.

Second-Degree Burn

This is also called a partial-thickness burn injury. It's called a partial-thickness injury, because in addition to the outer skin layer (epidermis), part of the inner skin layer (dermis) has also been damaged. Second-degree burns are bright red (like the color of red meat), moist, and painful to the touch. Many times they will also blister and look like an open wound. They generally take two to three weeks to heal.

Other information about second-degree burns:

- Seek medical care if it is a large wound. Consult a doctor if you're concerned.

- In very young or elderly patients, a second-degree burn (like a scald) can convert to a deeper and more serious burn.

- Second-degree burns become more serious when combined with other health problems.

- Second-degree burns to more than 10 percent of the body should be treated at a specialized burn center. If the area is deep, sometimes skin grafting may be required.

Third-Degree Burn

This is also called a full-thickness burn injury. It's called a full-thickness burn injury because besides the outer skin layer (epidermis), the full inner skin layer (epidermis, dermis, and subcutaneous tissue) has also been damaged. The color of third-degree burns may vary: They look like an open wound that may be dark red (like the color of red wine), white, brown and leathery, or charred in appearance. They are less painful to the touch because the nerve endings have been damaged. Seek medical care for any third-degree burn.

Other information about third-degree burns:

- Surgery will be required for skin grafting unless it is a very small area.

- In the very young or with elderly patients, or those with other health problems or trauma, any burn can make the injury more serious.

- Third-degree burns should be treated at a specialized burn center.

Burns that require specialized care in a burn facility:

- Second-degree burns affecting more than 10 percent of the body surface.

- Any third-degree burn requires immediate medical care.

- Burns over sensitive areas like joints, face, head, neck, genitals, or hands, or where joint function or cosmetic outcome could be compromised.

- Electrical (including lightening), chemical burns, or inhalation injuries.

- Patients who also have serious health problems beside the burn injury.

- Patients who have trauma and burns should be evaluated by the physician. If the trauma is the greater threat to life, treatment initially at a trauma center is needed.

- Burned children need specialized burn care in facilities that have equipment and personnel trained to deal with the special needs of children.

Chapter 46

What You Should Know About Animal Bites

Animal bites can sometimes result in severe infections and some people are at higher risk than others. Are you at risk? And do you know what to do if you are bitten?

The information and recommendations here will help you avoid serious problems.

I've always heard that dogs' mouths are cleaner than humans. Is this true?

Neither dogs nor cats nor humans have mouths that can even remotely be considered clean. All are filled with bacteria, many of which can cause disease if they enter broken skin. Over 130 disease-causing microbes have been isolated from dog and cat bite wounds. Animals' saliva is also heavily contaminated with bacteria, so a bite may not even be necessary to cause infection; if you have a cut or scratch and allow a pet to lick it, you could be setting yourself up for trouble.

What are the particular dangers from animal bites?

Bites to the hand, whether from cats or dogs, are potentially dangerous because of the structure of the hand. There are many bones, tendons, and joints in the hand and there is less blood circulation in these areas. This makes it harder for the body to fight infection in the hand. Infections that develop in the hand may lead to severe complications, such as osteomyelitis or septic arthritis.

About This Chapter: Text in this chapter is from "What You Should Know About Animal Bites," reprinted with permission from Louisiana State University School of Veterinary Medicine (www.vetmed.lsu.edu), © 2009. All rights reserved.

In small children, bites to the face, neck, or head are extremely hazardous. Because their small stature often puts their heads near dogs' mouths, children are often bitten in these areas. Dog bites can cause fractures of the face and skull and lead to brain and nervous system infections. Dog bites cause, on average, about 15–20 fatalities a year in the United States. Most of these victims are infants and young children.

Which is worse, dog bites or cat bites?

Dogs have strong jaws—large dogs can exert more than 450 pounds of pressure per square inch—and their teeth are relatively dull.

So the wounds caused by dogs are usually crushing of the tissue bitten and lacerations or tearing of the skin rather than puncture wounds. Most dog bites do not penetrate deeply enough to get bacteria into bones, tendons, or joints, but they often do a lot of damage just from the trauma of the bite. Tissue that has been crushed, however, such as may occur with a bite to the hand, is particularly susceptible to infection.

Cats' teeth are thin and sharp, so the wounds they cause are more likely to be puncture wounds. These wounds can reach into joints and bones and introduce bacteria deeply into the tissue. Puncture wounds are very difficult to clean, so a lot of bacteria may be left in the wound. Also, most cat bites are to the hand, which makes infection more likely.

Dog bites often do more outright damage, but only 3 to 18 percent become infected. In contrast, cat bites may appear more trivial, but up to 80 percent of cat bites may become infected if proper care is not taken.

What kinds of infections can develop?

Many infection-causing bacteria have been isolated from dog and cat bite wounds. The four we discuss here are probably the most significant.

Pasteurellosis: The most common bite-associated infection is caused by a bacterium called *Pasteurella*. Most cats and dogs—even healthy ones—naturally carry this organism in their mouths. When an animal bites a person (or another animal), these bacteria can enter the wound and start an infection. The first signs of pasteurellosis usually occur within two to twelve hours of the bite and include pain, reddening, and swelling of the area around the site of the bite. Pasteurellosis can progress quickly, spreading toward the body from the bitten area. It is important that you seek medical care immediately if these symptoms occur. Untreated, this infection can lead to severe complications. Bites to the hand need special attention; if pasteurellosis develops in the tissues of the hand, the bacteria can infect tendons or even bones and sometimes cause permanent damage if appropriate medical care is not administered promptly.

Streptococcal And Staphylococcal Infections: These bacteria can cause infections similar to those caused by *Pasteurella*. Redness and painful swelling occur at or near the site of the bite and progress toward the body. As with pasteurellosis, you should seek prompt medical care if these symptoms develop.

Capnocytophaga Infection: This is a very rare infection, but we mention it here because it is so dangerous if it develops. There is no common name for this infection, which is caused by the bacterium *Capnocytophaga canimorsus*. Most of the people who have become infected were bitten by dogs; in many instances the bite wounds themselves were tiny and would not have ordinarily called for any special medical care. But *Capnocytophaga* can cause septicemia, or blood poisoning, particularly in people whose immune systems are compromised by some underlying condition (see box). Up to 30 percent of people who have developed this septicemia have died. People who have had their spleens removed are at special risk for this infection. Early symptoms may include nausea, headache, muscle aches, and tiny reddened patches on the skin.

Underlying Conditions

If you have any of the risk factors listed below, particularly if you have had your spleen removed, it is very important that you take proper immediate care of any animal bite wound and promptly seek medical advice.

How do I know if I am at risk for infection?

Anyone who is bitten by a cat or a dog and who does not take proper care of the wound is at risk of developing infection. But some people are at increased risk.

- Are you over 50 years of age?
- Do you have diabetes, circulatory problems, liver disease, alcoholism, or HIV/AIDS?
- Have you had a mastectomy or organ transplant?
- Are you taking chemotherapy or long-term steroids?
- Have you had your spleen removed?

If you answered "yes" to any of these questions, you may be more likely to develop a serious infection than other people. You should take special care to avoid being bitten or scratched by any animal.

What should I do if I am bitten?

Immediately and thoroughly wash the wound with plenty of soap and warm water. The idea is to remove as much dirt and saliva—and therefore, bacteria—as possible. It may hurt to scrub a wound, but an infection will hurt a lot more. Scrub it well and run water over it for several minutes to make sure it is clean and all soap is rinsed out. It is a good idea to follow the washing with an antiseptic solution, such as iodine or other disinfectant, but always wash with soap and water first. Apply antibiotic ointment and cover the wound with gauze or a bandage. If the wound is severe, or if you have any of the risk factors listed above, seek medical advice at once. Your doctor may want you to take antibiotics to prevent infection from developing. If you have not had a recent tetanus booster, you may be advised to take one. And if you are bitten by a wild or stray animal that could have rabies, you may need to begin anti-rabies treatment.

If you have had your spleen removed, you should be aware that the potential for fatal infection exists, even from seemingly minor wounds. Some experts recommend that people without spleens should completely avoid contact with cats and dogs. This is an issue you and your doctor should discuss in detail.

For most people, however, the benefits of companion animals outweigh the risk. If you have any of the risk factors shown in the box above, you should do everything possible to avoid being bitten or scratched by dogs or cats. If wounds do occur, you should clean them promptly and thoroughly and seek medical advice. A little care and common sense can go a long way in preventing bite-associated infections.

If you are bitten by any animal, always consult your physician for his/her recommendations.

Chapter 47

Insect Bites And Stings

Bug bites and stings are, for the most part, no more unpleasant than a homework assignment—kind of annoying but basically harmless. Occasionally, though, an insect bite or sting can cause serious problems. You should know when a simple ice pack can bring some relief or when a visit to the local hospital is in order.

Before you find out how to handle your unwelcome guests, come meet the critters who want a little piece of you.

Bee And Wasp Stings

For most people, being stung by a bee is a minor nuisance. The affected area may get a little red or swollen and it may be slightly painful, but that's about it.

Bee and wasp stings can cause real problems for people who are allergic, though. A person can get a localized allergic reaction (swelling, heat, or itching of the skin around the bite area) or a **systemic** allergic reaction, meaning that the poison causes a reaction throughout a person's body, not just around the bite area.

In the case of a systemic reaction, the person may break out in hives. Other symptoms include wheezing; shortness of breath; rapid heartbeat; faintness; and swelling of the face, lips, or tongue. If a person has these symptoms, it's important to get help immediately. It hardly ever happens, but severe allergic reactions to bee stings can be fatal if the person doesn't get medical help.

About This Chapter: "Bug Bites And Stings," May 2010, reprinted with permission from www.kidshealth.org. This information was provided by KidsHealth®, one of the largest resources online for medically reviewed health information written for parents, kids, and teens. For more articles like this, visit www.KidsHealth.org, or www.TeensHealth.org. Copyright © 1995-2012 The Nemours Foundation. All rights reserved.

Flea And Tick Bites

Fleas can be lumped into the irritating-but-not-serious category as well. They are often found on Fido or Fluffy, but they can also be attracted to you.

Depending on where you live, **ticks** could ruin a good camping trip. One variety known as deer ticks is known to carry Lyme disease, so the trick is to get them off your body fast. In the United States, the northeastern and upper midwestern states are most affected by the threat of disease from ticks, but some cases have been found in the Pacific Northwest and in northern and southern Europe. Ticks can carry other diseases, too, such as Rocky Mountain spotted fever. Ticks are usually found in heavily wooded areas.

Mosquito Bites

Mosquitoes hang out anywhere people, food, or pools of still water are found. Generally they aren't anything to worry about: They bite, you itch, end of story.

However, there is some concern about West Nile virus, which is transmitted to humans by mosquitoes. The good news is that healthy kids, teens, and adults under 50 are at low risk of catching West Nile virus. And although the virus can put people at risk for developing a serious infection called encephalitis, in reality this hardly ever happens. Less than 1 percent of the people who are infected with West Nile virus become seriously ill.

Spider Bites

Most spider bites are minor, although they can cause mild swelling or allergic reactions. But a small percentage of teens become ill after being bitten by brown recluse or black widow spiders. Although not everyone will have a reaction, you should see a doctor and get treatment quickly if you know you've been bitten by one of these spiders.

The **brown recluse** is brown (big surprise) with a small shape of a violin in a darker brown area on the back of its head. These spiders are small but tough: a half-inch body (about 1 centimeter) with legs stretching another inch (3 centimeters) or even more. They are found mostly in midwestern and southern parts of the United States, and they like to hide in dark, quiet places like attics or garages. When humans enter their space unexpectedly, they bite out of fear. The bites usually don't hurt at first—and most people don't even know that they've been bitten.

Brown recluse bites don't cause problems for most people. But in a small percentage of cases, they can lead to skin damage and scarring. The few people who do have a reaction may notice swelling and skin changes 4 to 8 hours after the bite. The swelling may form a blister. If this happens, a dark, scabby material called eschar (pronounced: **es**-kar) may cover the blister within a week after the bite. Most brown recluse bites get better on their own—but it can take a couple of months. So it's always a good idea to see a doctor for proper treatment.

The **black widow** is found in southern Canada, throughout the United States, and in Mexico. Easily identified by its shiny coal-black body and orange hourglass shape on its underbelly, it's a similar size to the brown recluse spider and it should be treated as carefully.

Most often, people who have been bitten by a black widow don't even know it until they feel the symptoms. But the good news is that there are lots of warning signs that give you time to act before things get too serious. The venom (poison) in a black widow bite causes a systemic reaction.

Someone who has been bitten by a black widow may get painful cramps within a few hours. These cramps usually make a person feel achy all over, and can spread to include abdominal cramping, which may be severe. The person may also have nausea, vomiting, chills, fever, and headache. If you show any of these symptoms, get to the hospital immediately.

Spider bites can sound scary, but it's actually extremely rare that a person will die from one. Fewer than 1 percent of the people who report being bitten by a black widow die, and even fewer people die from brown recluse bites. Young children are most at risk.

What To Do

For most varieties of bug bites and stings, antihistamines will help to stop itching and lessen swelling, and acetaminophen can help relieve any pain. Ibuprofen can help reduce swelling while relieving some pain. Some people use a topical 1% hydrocortisone cream (sold in pharmacies without a prescription) to alleviate itching.

Say goodbye to ticks by removing them with a pair of tweezers as soon as you notice them. Ticks removed within 24 to 48 hours are less likely to transmit diseases like Lyme disease. Be sure to pull a tick out from the head, which is closest to your skin, to ensure that you remove the whole thing. Have someone help you get the hard-to-reach places of your body, and pull each one out very slowly. Clean the site with soap and water, and treat with an antiseptic or antibiotic cream to avoid infection.

Do not try to burn a tick off, as the flame only agitates the insect, causing it to burrow deeper into your skin. When you've pulled the tick out, put it in a jar of rubbing alcohol to kill it. (Your doctor may also want you to save the tick so that its type can be identified.)

After a bee sting, if you can see the stinger, remove it as quickly as possible to lessen your exposure to the venom.

Wash the sting or bite with soap and water and keep it clean. Apply some calamine lotion or a paste of water and baking soda (unless the sting is near your eyes). Put an ice pack on the affected area for 15 minutes every few hours or so, or cover the sting with a cold compress. Apply an antibiotic cream to prevent further infection. Using a 1% hydrocortisone cream can reduce redness, swelling, itching, and pain.

If you are allergic to bee stings, see your doctor for a prescription for an epinephrine kit. If used immediately after a bee attack, this shot will stop the allergic reaction before it starts, which could save your life. An epinephrine kit is easy to use—your doctor or pharmacist will explain how.

If you're severely allergic to bug bites and stings, talk to a doctor about getting venom immunotherapy (shots) from an allergist.

Serious Stuff—Seek Medical Help

How do you know when a sting or bite is too much for you to handle alone? If you have any symptoms of a systemic allergic reaction, get to the emergency department right away. These symptoms include:

- shortness of breath
- wheezing
- redness or hives over most of your body
- swelling of the face, lips, or tongue
- feeling like your throat is closing up
- nausea
- vomiting
- chills
- muscle aches or cramps
- weakness
- fever

In the case of a black widow spider bite, or if you have any doubt about what kind of spider bit you and you're feeling sick and have cramps, get to the emergency department immediately. (Take the spider with you if you were able to kill it safely.)

If bites or stings get infected or if an open sore or blister refuses to heal, make an appointment with your family doctor.

Preventing Bites And Stings

Human beings don't have to sit around and wait to be a sample on the insect buffet. Here are some steps we can take to protect ourselves:

- Prevent flea infestations by treating your house (including all carpets, furniture, and pets) regularly during the warmer months. Frequent vacuuming can also help.

- Avoid mosquitoes by staying away from areas where mosquitoes breed, such as still pools or ponds, during hot weather. Remove standing water from birdbaths, buckets, etc.; try to stay inside when mosquitoes are most active (dawn and dusk); and wear insect repellent when you are outside.

- When in tick country, take turns with friends and family checking one another for ticks every few hours. Remove any you find immediately. The most important places to check are behind your ears, on your scalp, on the back of your neck, in your armpits, in your groin area, and behind your knees. If you have a pet with you, check your pet, too! Use tick products on pets to prevent them from being bitten.

- Use insect repellent when spending time outdoors camping, hiking, or on the beach. Repellents that contain 10% to 30% DEET (N,N-diethyl-meta-toluamide) are approved for mosquitoes, ticks, and some other bugs. Repellents that contain picaridin (KBR 3023) or oil of lemon eucalyptus (p-menthane 3,8-diol or PMD) are effective against mosquitoes. Follow the instructions carefully and don't overuse the product—using more than you need won't give you any extra protection. Reapply insect repellent after swimming or if you've been sweating for a long time.

- When you are in wooded areas, tuck your clothes in and try to keep as covered up as possible. Tuck pants into socks, shirts into pants, and sleeves into gloves. Wear shoes and socks when walking on grass, even it's just for a minute. Bees and wasps can sting your unprotected feet.

- Wear gloves if you're gardening.

- Don't disturb bee or wasp nests.

- Don't swat at buzzing insects—they will sting if they feel threatened.

- Be aware that spiders might be hiding in undisturbed piles of wood, seldom-opened boxes, or corners behind furniture, and proceed with caution.

Chapter 48

Poison Ivy, Poison Oak, And Poison Sumac

A walk in the woods is a wonderful outdoor activity. Contact with a patch of poison ivy, oak, or sumac is not.

Learning to recognize these plants and staying away from them is the best form of treatment. Contact with the green or dried parts of any of the plants can cause an uncomfortable, itchy rash that has a streaked or spotted appearance.

Cause

The poison ivy rash is actually an allergic reaction to the plant oil. As with all allergies, not all people will develop the same reaction. All parts of the plant contain the oil. Dried leaves and stems can bring about a reaction as can the smoke from burning plants, so take care when burning brush or lighting campfires. Contrary to popular belief, drainage from the blisters cannot spread a poison ivy rash. Only the plant oil causes the reaction. Open blisters can become infected, though, so keep the area clean. Dogs and other animals don't seem to be affected by poison ivy, but they can carry the oil on their fur and cause a reaction in people who touch the fur. Other ways the oil can be carried are on shoes, toys, clothing, and even golf balls that have gone through the rough. The severity of your reaction can change over a period of time, too. Highly sensitive people can become resistant, while others who have never had a prior reaction can suddenly develop a nasty case of poison ivy.

About This Chapter: Reprinted with permission from "Poison Ivy," part of the Tips to Grow By™ series produced as a public service of Akron Children's Hospital. Copyright ©2009 Akron Children's Hospital. For additional information, visit https://www.akronchildrens.org/cms/tips_to_grow_by/index.html.

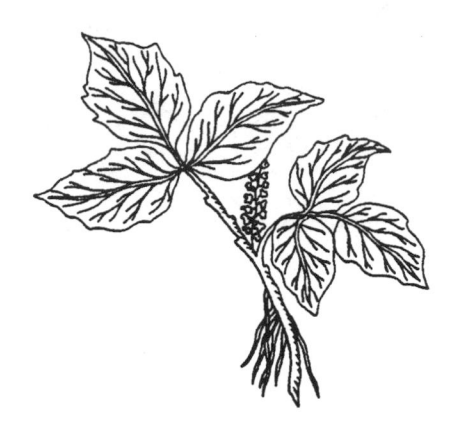

Figure 48.1. Poison Ivy

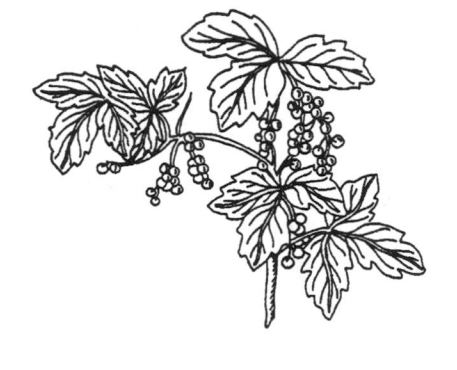

Figure 48.2. Poison Oak

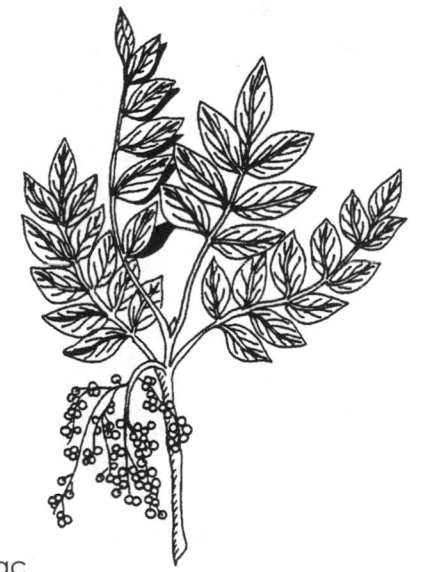

Figure 48.3. Poison Sumac

Symptoms

You'll first notice redness, swelling, and itching at the site about two days after contact. After a few days, blisters can form in a streaked or spotted rash, oozing a serum from damaged skin cells. The lesions will dry, heal, and stop itching in 10 to 14 days.

Treatment

If you know you have come in contact with one of the poisonous plants, wash the exposed skin with soap and water for at least 10 minutes to remove the plant oil. Use care with clothing—the oil can spread from the clothes to the skin and cause a new or wider rash. Wash all clothing promptly and thoroughly. There are several ways to increase comfort when a case of poison ivy develops. Cool compresses, calamine lotion applied to the rash with a cotton ball, and oatmeal baths are all time-honored treatments. Topical corticosteroid ointment is effective for the prevention or relief of inflammation, especially when applied before blisters appear.

When To Call The Doctor

Call your doctor if you have:

*   A rash on more than one-fourth of the body

*   Poison ivy on the face, lips, eyes or genitals

*   Signs of infection: a sore and tender rash rather than an itchy one; increased redness; yellow drainage from the blisters; and/or a fever

Prevention

The best way to prevent poison ivy rashes is to avoid the plants that cause these allergic reactions. Learn to recognize these plants. Poison ivy grows almost everywhere east of the Rocky Mountains. Poison oak is mainly found west of the Rockies, and poison sumac is usually restricted to swamp areas in the southeast. The only areas of the country where there is little likelihood of finding these plants are areas above 4,000 feet in elevation; and Nevada, Hawaii, and Alaska.

Chapter 49

Frostbite

Introduction

Frostbite is damage to skin and tissue caused by exposure to freezing temperatures—typically any temperature below minus 0.55° C (31° F).

Frostbite can affect any part of your body. However, the extremities—such as the hands, feet, ears, nose, and lips—are most likely to be affected.

The symptoms of frostbite are varied, but usually begin with the affected parts feeling cold and painful. If exposure to the cold continues, you may feel pins and needles before the area becomes numb as the tissues freeze.

The severity of frostbite and how quickly it develops depends on how cold it is and the length of exposure.

The effects of frostbite range from minor tissue damage that fully recovers without treatment to severe tissue loss that requires surgery or even amputation to remove dead tissues.

If you think you or someone else may have frostbite, call your family doctor for advice.

If the symptoms are more severe, go immediately to your nearest accident and emergency department.

Symptoms Of Frostbite

The symptoms of frostbite progress in stages. The longer the body is exposed to freezing conditions and the colder the temperature is, the more advanced frostbite can become.

About This Chapter: "Frostbite—Introduction," and "Frostbite—Symptoms," reprinted from NHS Choices, www.nhs.uk. Reproduced by kind permission of the Department of Health, © 2013.

What's It Mean?

Extremities: Hands, feet, ears, nose, and lips—parts of body most vulnerable to frostbite.

Frostnip: First stage of frostbite involving feeling of pins and needles, numbness, tingling, or aching.

Hypothermia: Life-threatening drop in body temperature.

Superficial Frostbite: Intermediate frostbite stage involving hard, frozen feeling of affected area followed by redness, blisters, and pain on thawing.

Tissue Necrosis: When part of the skin or surrounding tissue has died.

—LE

Early Stage—Frostnip

During the early stage of frostbite, you will have pins and needles, throbbing, or aching in the affected area. The skin will become cold, numb, and white, and you may feel a tingling sensation.

This stage of frostbite is also known as frostnip, and is common in people who live or work in cold climates. The extremities, such as the fingers, nose, ears, and toes, are most commonly affected.

Intermediate Stage

After these early signs, prolonged exposure to cold temperatures will cause more tissue damage. The affected area will feel hard and frozen. When you are out of the cold and the tissue is thawed out, the skin will turn red and blister, which can be painful. There may also be swelling and itching.

This is known as superficial frostbite because it affects the top layers of skin and tissue. The skin underneath the blisters is usually still intact but treatment is needed to make sure there is no lasting damage.

Advanced Stage

When exposure to the cold continues, frostbite becomes increasingly severe. The skin becomes white, blue, or blotchy, and the tissue underneath feels hard and cold to touch. There may be further damage to tendons, muscles, nerves, and bones beneath the skin.

This is known as deep frostbite and requires urgent medical attention.

As the skin thaws, blood-filled blisters form and turn into thick black scabs. At this stage, it is likely that some tissue has died. This is known as tissue necrosis, and the tissue may have to be removed to prevent infection.

Long-Term Effects

People with a history of severe frostbite often report further long-term effects of frostbite. These can include:

- Increased sensitivity to cold

- Numbness in the affected body parts, most commonly the fingers

- Reduced sense of touch in the affected body part

- Persistent pain in the affected body part

Treating Frostbite

It is important that a person with frostbite is taken to a warm environment as soon as it is safe to do so, as they are also likely to have hypothermia. Do not put pressure on the frostbitten area.

The affected area should be re-warmed slowly by immersing it in warm (but not hot) water. However, do this only if there is no possibility of further freezing. If re-warmed tissue becomes frozen again, there will be further tissue damage.

A bath of water at 40° C–41° C (104° F–105.8° F) is recommended for re-warming. This process may be very painful and large amounts of painkillers are often required. Ideally, re-warming should be performed by trained medical professionals.

Preventing Frostbite

Almost all cases of frostbite can be prevented by:

- Wearing appropriate clothing: Multiple layers of warm, loose clothing are better than a single layer.

- Wearing a weatherproof hat that covers your ears: A surprising amount of heat can be lost through your head.

- Avoiding unnecessary exposure to cold.

- Keeping dry: Remove any wet clothing.

- Planning for emergencies: For example making sure you keep a warm blanket and some spare clothes if driving in icy conditions in case you break down.

Who's At Risk Of Frostbite?

Certain groups of people are at greater risk of getting frostbite. They include:

- People who take part in winter and high-altitude sports, such mountaineers and skiers

- Anyone stranded in extreme cold weather conditions

- Anyone with a job that means they are outdoors in harsh conditions for a long time, such as soldiers, sailors, and rescue workers

- Homeless people

- The very young and very old, as their bodies are less able to regulate body temperature

- People with conditions that cause blood vessel damage or circulation problems, such as diabetes and Raynaud's phenomenon

- Anyone taking medications that constrict the blood vessels, including beta blockers (smoking can also constrict the blood vessels)

Many cases of frostbite occur in people who have taken drugs or drunk alcohol and who fall asleep outside in cold weather.

As you would expect, cases of frostbite in England often rise during particularly cold winters. For example, during the very cold winter of 2010–2011, there were 111 hospital admissions for frostbite. In most years, there are only around 30–60 cases every winter.

Complications

Complications of frostbite can be serious and include:

- A life-threatening drop in body temperature (hypothermia)

- The affected body part becoming particularly vulnerable to infections, such as tetanus

- Long-term pain

Chapter 50

Corns And Calluses

Corns and calluses are thickened layers of skin caused by repeated pressure or friction.

Causes

Corns and calluses are caused by pressure or friction on skin. A corn is thickened skin on the top or side of a toe, usually from shoes that do not fit properly. A callus is thickened skin on your hands or the soles of your feet.

The thickening of the skin is a protective reaction. For example, farmers and rowers get callused hands that prevent them from getting painful blisters. People with bunions often develop a callus over the bunion because it rubs against the shoe.

Neither corns nor calluses are serious conditions.

Symptoms

- Skin is thick and hardened.

- Skin may be flaky and dry.

- Hardened, thick skin areas are found on hands, feet, or other areas that may be rubbed or pressed.

Exams And Tests

Your health care provider will make the diagnosis after observing the skin. In most cases tests are not necessary.

About This Chapter: "Corns and Calluses," © 2013 A.D.A.M., Inc. Reprinted with permission.

Treatment

Usually, preventing friction is the only treatment needed. If a corn is the result of a poor-fitting shoe, changing to shoes that fit properly will usually eliminate the corn within a couple of weeks. Until then, protect the skin with donut-shaped corn pads, available in pharmacies. If desired, use a pumice stone to gently wear down the corn.

Calluses on the hands can be treated by wearing gloves during activities that cause friction, such as gardening and weightlifting.

If an infection or ulcer occurs in an area of a callus or corn, unhealthy tissue may need to be removed by a health care provider and treatment with antibiotics may be necessary.

Calluses often reflect undue pressure placed on the skin because of an underlying problem such as bunions. Proper treatment of any underlying condition should prevent the calluses from returning.

Outlook (Prognosis)

Corns and calluses are rarely serious. If treated properly, they should improve without causing long-term problems.

Possible Complications

Complications of corns and calluses are rare. People with diabetes are prone to ulcers and infections and should regularly examine their feet to identify any problems right away. Such foot injuries need medical attention.

When To Contact A Medical Professional

Very closely check your feet if you have diabetes or numbness in the feet or toes. If you have diabetes and notice problems with your feet, contact your health care provider.

Otherwise, simply changing to better-fitting shoes or wearing gloves should resolve most problems with corns and calluses.

If you suspect that your corn or callus is infected or is not getting better despite treatment, contact your health care provider. Also call your health care provider if you have continued symptoms of pain, redness, warmth, or drainage.

Alternative Names

Calluses and corns.

Chapter 51

Skin Picking

What is chronic skin picking?

Chronic skin picking (CSP) is a serious and poorly understood problem. People who suffer from CSP repetitively touch, rub, scratch, pick at, or dig into their skin, often in an attempt to remove small irregularities or perceived imperfections. This behavior may result in skin discoloration or scarring. In more serious cases, severe tissue damage and visible disfigurement can result.

CSP is now thought of as one of many body-focused repetitive behaviors (BFRBs) in which a person can cause harm or damage to themselves or their appearance. Other BFRBs include chronic hair pulling (trichotillomania), biting the insides of the cheeks, and severe nail biting.

Skin picking or other BFRBs can occur when a person experiences feelings such as anxiety, fear, excitement or boredom. Some people report that the act of repetitively picking at their skin is pleasurable. Many hours can be spent picking the skin, and this repetitive behavior can negatively impact a person's social, work, and family relationships.

Though skin picking often occurs on its own—unconnected to other physical or mental disorders—it is important to identify whether or not skin picking is a symptom of another problem that needs treatment. For example, skin picking could be a symptom of illnesses such as dermatological disorders, autoimmune problems, body dysmorphic disorder, obsessive-compulsive disorder, substance abuse disorders (such as opiate withdrawal), developmental disorders (like autism), and psychosis. Establishing whether skin picking is an independent problem or a symptom of another disorder is an important first step in creating an appropriate treatment plan.

About This Chapter: From "Skin Picking: Frequently Asked Questions," © 2012 Trichotillomania Learning Center, Inc. (www.trich.org). Reprinted with permission.

Am I the only one who picks my skin?

No, most people pick their skin to some degree. Occasional picking at cuticles, acne blemishes, scabs, calluses, or other skin irregularities is a very common human behavior. It also is not unusual for skin picking to actually become a problem, whether temporary or chronic. In fact, studies indicate that 2 percent of all dermatology patients and 4 percent of college students pick their skin to the point where it causes noticeable tissue damage and marked distress or impairment in daily functioning. It is important to remember that you are not alone with this problem.

When is skin picking a serious problem?

There is no universally agreed-upon standard as to when skin picking becomes a serious problem. In more serious cases, though, the picking is generally time-consuming, results in noticeable tissue damage, and causes emotional distress. When it is even more severe, people often suffer impairment in social, occupational, and physical functioning. This can include avoiding social activities such as going to the pool, gym, or beach; being late for work or other events because of the time it takes to cover up the picking; and avoiding contact with anyone who may notice bleeding, scars, or sores.

What causes chronic skin picking?

The cause of this disorder remains a mystery. However, research shows that some animals also pick or chew at their bodies, causing great damage. Because of this similarity, and the fact that in some women skin picking can fluctuate with the menstrual cycle, many believe that skin picking has an underlying genetic or biological cause.

Skin picking may also serve as an emotional outlet for some people. Repetitive skin picking appears to be a way for some people to increase their activity levels when they are bored, or to control their emotions when they are feeling anxious, tense, or upset. The fact that some individuals can actually regulate their emotions by picking their skin may be why they develop this problem in the first place. Skin picking may cause a person to "numb" or "zone out" as a way of dealing with feelings that seem overwhelming. However, this has not been scientifically proven.

Is skin-picking a self-injurious behavior, like cutting or burning yourself?

No. Chronic skin picking can sometimes be confused with self-injurious and self-mutilating behaviors like cutting or burning of the skin because of the appearance of skin wounds and the fact that skin picking is self-inflicted. However, it is very important to distinguish between these two types of behaviors. People with CSP do not wish to cause themselves pain in order to relieve a sense of numbness or to assert a level of control over their bodies like those who cut or burn themselves. While people who pick their skin may find picking to be a pleasurable act, the aftermath is actually one of distress and remorse.

How does chronic skin picking start?

Skin picking can begin in a number of ways, but two in particular are quite common. First, a person may experience an injury to or disease of the skin. When the wound starts to heal, a scab forms and sometimes starts to itch. This may lead the person to pick or scratch at the scab. Unfortunately, with further trauma, the skin never completely heals. This can result in repeated scabbing and itching, which is then relieved with further picking. In other cases, people with chronic skin picking report that picking began during, or soon after, a very stressful event in their lives. The person slowly learns that skin picking can work to control their feelings and emotions and they continue to pick in the future.

At what age do people usually start picking?

The behavior can begin at any age, from preteen to older adult, and last for months or years. How the disorder progresses depends on many factors, including the stresses in a person's life, and whether or not the person seeks and finds appropriate treatment.

Why does skin picking become a problem for some people and not for others?

A large number of people habitually pick their skin, but it only becomes a severe problem for a relatively small number of people. The reasons for this are unclear, but one school of thought is that some people have a genetic or biological predisposition and thus are more likely to develop CSP. A second possibility is that those who develop a skin picking problem experience greater levels of anxiety, stress, or boredom than those who do not.

Am I damaging my skin when I pick?

A number of things can happen when you pick your skin. While it is possible that you will not cause any permanent damage, in some cases an infection can develop in the area that was picked. You can tell that your skin has become infected if it is red, warm, and tender. (If this red, warm, and tender area does not heal quickly or begins to grow and spread from its initial location, you should seek medical treatment for the infection.)

Repeated skin picking also can cause the skin at the picking site to change color when it heals. It may take many months for the skin to return to its normal color and this will only happen if the spot is not picked. But it is also possible that the skin will remain permanently discolored.

You can get scars from repetitive skin picking. Scars can occur if you pick all the way through the top layer of the skin, called the epidermis, down into the next skin layer, called the dermis, or beyond. Picking this deep removes melanin, the pigment that gives skin its color. Most scars are small, but extensive; deep skin picking can lead to visible scars or uneven skin texture that will not go away.

Is help available?

Yes, help is available for chronic skin picking, but it can be hard to find. Since CSP is still a largely misunderstood problem, few medical and mental health professionals are adequately trained to treat the behavior successfully. However, as chronic skin picking becomes a more recognized and understood problem, more professionals are becoming familiar with interventions that can help. The Trichotillomania Learning Center (TLC) keeps a database of treatment professionals who are knowledgeable about this disorder and can help you in your search for a local treatment provider.

Psychologists and therapists who specialize in cognitive-behavioral therapy, which addresses both the thoughts of an individual and their behaviors, are good resources for skin picking problems. Dermatologists or psychiatrists can also prescribe medications that may help to eliminate skin irritations or reduce urges to pick, but results vary widely. Either option (or both) may prove useful depending upon your needs and personal approach to treatment.

What is the treatment and is it effective?

The primary treatment approach for CSP is a form of cognitive-behavioral therapy called **habit reversal training (HRT)**. Over the years, HRT has been expanded to become a comprehensive approach to understanding the physical and emotional triggers, situational factors, and associated behaviors involved in problems like chronic skin picking. Once these factors are understood, alternative coping strategies are taught. This includes instruction in competing motor responses that actually prevent you from picking—for example, keeping your hands busy by holding and squeezing a rubber ball whenever you feel the urge to pick at your skin.

Another approach to treatment is called **stimulus control (SC),** which involves modifying physical aspects of a skin picker's environment to reduce sensory input that leads to picking.

For example, if looking closely at your skin in the bathroom mirror causes you to pick your face, then the sensory input of seeing your pores needs to be modified. Try putting a piece of tape on the floor to remind you not to get too close to the mirror. If just touching your skin is a trigger for you, you might wear gloves, Band-Aids, or rubber fingertips to prevent you from feeling your skin and help you resist the urge to pick. Or you might be instructed to avoid or alter situations that are high risk to you, such as sitting for long periods of time reading or using the computer. Overall, it is important to recognize that skin picking can be a complex problem and might need to be approached from several different angles to treat it properly.

Although few studies have been conducted to assess the effectiveness of these treatments, several case studies and small investigations support the use of HRT and SC for skin picking. In addition, there is some research support for the use of certain medications known as selective serotonin reuptake inhibitors (SSRIs), including fluoxetine, fluvoxamine, sertraline, paroxetine, citalopram, and escitalopram. Additionally, preliminary research indicates that the effectiveness of certain medications in reducing impulses for specific behaviors (such as alcohol abuse) may also be useful in treating CSP.

Where can I find help?

If you are concerned with any medical aspects of your skin picking—a wound that may be infected, for example, or lesions that have not healed over time—it is important to first consult with your primary care physician or a dermatologist. (Do not be alarmed if your doctor is not familiar with CSP; you may have to educate him or her about your skin picking and its impact on you.) After any medical concerns are addressed, it is recommended that you seek help from a psychologist or therapist who can work with you to develop a behavioral program to address your chronic skin picking. TLC provides listings of treatment providers.

It also is important to determine the level of experience and the treatment approach of any professional you plan to go to for help. When interviewing a potential treatment provider, ask if he or she has specific training in treating body-focused repetitive behavior (BFRB) problems such as skin picking. Ask them to describe their treatment approach to you, and listen for terms like "cognitive-behavioral therapy," "habit reversal training," and "stimulus control." Self-education and self-help are also options for people who are unable to locate trained professionals; TLC (www.trich.org) can provide additional information and help in locating or starting self-help support groups in your area.

If your insurance company does not have professionals trained to treat this problem, request that they provide out-of- network coverage for providers with this training. Insurance companies are required to make exceptions when they cannot provide services within their panel of providers. Ideally, you will want to find a professional who is trained specifically in cognitive-behavioral therapy for BFRBs.

If you are unable to find someone trained in BFRB treatment in your area, you may need to find a professional who is experienced with behavior therapy and willing to learn more about skin picking. Professionals trained in the treatment of obsessive-compulsive disorder are also often familiar with behavior therapy for conditions like chronic skin picking and may be well positioned to adapt their skills to help with BFRBs.

Chapter 52

Nail Abnormalities

Introduction

Fingernail or toenail abnormalities can tell you a lot about your health. They're often a sign of a fungal nail infection or injury, but can sometimes indicate a more serious underlying disease.

Visit your family doctor if your nails have obviously changed in color, texture, shape, or thickness and you don't know why (you haven't injured your nails or been biting them).

This chapter gives the most likely reasons for the following nail problems:

- Brittle or crumbly nails

- Discolored nails

- White nails

- Thickened, overgrown nails

- Loose nails

- Indented spoon-shaped nails

- Pitting or dents on the nails

- Grooves going across the width of the nails

- Unusually curved fingertips and nails

About This Chapter: Reprinted from NHS Choices, www.nhs.uk. Reproduced by kind permission of the Department of Health, © 2013.

- White lines running across the nails

- Dark stripes running down the nail

- Red or brown little streaks under the nails

- A destroyed nail

- Infected nail fold (painful, red, and swollen skin next to the nail)

Brittle Or Crumbly Nails

Brittle nails are often just a sign of ageing or long-term exposure to water or chemicals such as detergents and nail polish. Nails can be strengthened by taking biotin (vitamin B7) supplements, by wearing gloves for all wet work and by frequently applying moisturizing cream to the nails.

But sometimes, brittle or crumbly nails can be caused by:

- A fungal nail infection, which can be cleared by taking a course of antifungal tablets (this especially tends to be the cause of crumbly toenails)

- A skin condition called lichen planus, which can just affect the nails

- An underactive thyroid or overactive thyroid, where the thyroid gland in your neck either doesn't produce enough hormones or produces too many

- Nail psoriasis, a long-term skin condition that can cause the nails to become crumbly

A less common cause of crumbly nails is reactive arthritis, an unusual reaction of the immune system affecting the joints, muscles, and other parts of the body following an infection. If you have a combination of symptoms affecting different organs, your family doctor might consider this condition.

Discolored Nails

The most common cause of a yellow toenail is a fungal nail infection. Yellow nails can also result from any of the following:

- Frequent application of nail varnish (polish)

- Nail psoriasis (a common cause)

- Lymphedema, a long-term condition that causes swelling of the skin

- Permanent damage to your airways caused by bronchiectasis (a long-term lung condition)

- Sinusitis (inflammation of the lining of the sinuses)

- Inflammation of the thyroid gland in the neck

- Tuberculosis (TB), a bacterial infection that affects the lungs

- Jaundice (yellowing of the skin) due to liver disease

- Some drugs, such as mepacrine or carotene

- Chronic paronychia (infection of the nail fold)

Greenish-black nails can be caused by overgrowth of bacteria called *pseudomonas,* especially under loose nails. This can be treated by soaking the affected nails in an antiseptic solution or vinegar.

Gray nails can be caused by drugs such as antimalarials or minocycline.

Brown nails can sometimes be caused by thyroid disease, pregnancy, malnutrition, and exposure to chemicals such as nail polish.

Red Or Yellow Drop Under The Nail

If the discoloration looks like a drop of oil under the nail plate or is the color of salmon, you may have the skin condition psoriasis.

Half White, Half Brown Nails

Fingernails that are half white and half brown (brown near the tips) can be a sign of kidney failure, where the kidneys stop working properly. The link is not fully understood, but one theory is that kidney failure causes chemical changes in the blood that encourage melanin (a skin pigment) to be released into the nail bed. It's also possible that kidney failure causes an increase in the number of tiny blood vessels in the nail bed.

It is estimated that up to 40 percent of people with kidney failure have "half-and-half" fingernails.

Half-and-half nails have also been seen in some people with AIDS and can be seen following chemotherapy.

White Nails

If most of the nail plate has turned white and it is not because the nail has become detached from the nail bed, it is likely to be either a fungal nail infection or a sign of decreased blood supply to the nail bed, known as "Terry's nails."

Terry's nails are typically white with reddened or dark tips and can be a sign of a wide range of medical conditions, including the following:

- Liver cirrhosis (scarring and damage to the liver): About 80 percent of people with cirrhosis have Terry's nails.

- Liver, kidney, or heart failure

- Diabetes

- An overactive thyroid (where the thyroid gland in your neck produces too many hormones)

- Malnutrition

Thickened, Overgrown Nails

A common cause of thickened nails is a fungal nail infection. This can also cause them to discolor and become crumbly (see above).

Other possible causes of thickened or overgrown nails are:

- Psoriasis, a long-term condition that tends to also cause red, flaky patches of skin

- Long-term pressure from shoes that are either too small or too narrow over the toes

- Reactive arthritis, where the immune system attacks the joints, muscles, and other parts of the body following an infection

Severely Overgrown Horn-Like Nails

Sometimes, the big toenails become so overgrown and thickened that they resemble claws and are almost impossible to cut with conventional nail clippers. This nail disorder is known as onychogryphosis ("ram's horn nails"), and is seen in older people or as a response to long-term pressure on the nails. Regular chiropody can help, but sometimes the nails need to be removed by a podiatrist or doctor.

Loose Nails

It's normal for a toenail to come loose and fall off after an injury to the toe. However, if you haven't injured your nail, a loose nail is often caused by over-manicuring the nails and cleaning under the nails with a sharp object.

Less commonly, it may be a sign of one of the below health conditions:

- A fungal nail infection

- Psoriasis of the nail: Psoriasis is a long-term condition that tends to also cause red, flaky patches of skin.

- Warts that cluster around the fingernail

- An overactive thyroid, which means the thyroid gland in the neck is producing too many hormones

- Sarcoidosis, a condition where small clumps of cells form in the organs and tissues of the body

- Amyloidosis, where protein builds up in the organs

- A problem with the connective tissue fibers in the body that support the organs and body tissues

- Poor circulation, for example caused by smoking or Raynaud's disease (where the skin of the fingers turns white as a response to cold)

- An allergic reaction to medicine (usually to a type of antibiotic) or nail cosmetics

A loose nail should be cut back to allow the nail to become reattached as it grows. You should not clean your nails with anything other than a soft nailbrush.

Indented Spoon-Shaped Nails (Koilonychia)

If your fingernails curve inwards like spoons (known medically as koilonychia), you may have one of the following disorders:

- Iron-deficiency anemia, which is a reduced number of red blood cells due to a lack of iron in the body (the main symptoms of iron-deficiency anemia are tiredness and a lack of energy)

- Hemochromatosis, where the body contains too much iron

- Raynaud's disease, a common condition that affects the blood supply to the fingers and toes, causing them to turn white

- Lupus erythematosus, an uncommon condition where the immune system attacks the body's cells, tissues and organs

Pitting Or Dents On The Nails

Pitting or small dents on the surface of your nails can be a sign of any of the below diseases:

- Psoriasis, a long-term condition that tends to also cause red, flaky patches of skin (10 percent to 50 percent of patients with psoriasis have pitted nails)

- Eczema, a long-term skin condition

- Reactive arthritis, where the immune system attacks the joints, muscles, and other parts of the body following an infection

- Alopecia areata, patches of hair loss that tend to come and go

Grooves Across The Fingernails (Beau's Lines)

Deep lines or grooves that go from left to right across the nail are known as Beau's lines. They may be a sign of:

- An illness that started a few months ago

- Chemotherapy

- A previous injury

- Previous exposure to extremely cold temperatures, if you have Raynaud's disease (a common condition affecting the blood supply to the fingers and toes)

Illness, injury, or cold temperatures can interrupt nail growth and cause nail grooves to form at the base of the nails. These grooves tend to only be noticed a few months later, when the nails have grown and the grooves have moved up the nails to become visible. It takes about 4–6 months for a fingernail to fully grow out, and 6–12 months for a toenail.

Unusually Curved Fingertips And Nails

Clubbing of the fingertips means the tissue beneath the nails thickens and the fingertips become rounded and bulbous. The fingernails curve over the rounded fingertips.

Clubbing is thought to result from increased blood flow to the fingertips. It can run in families and be entirely harmless. However, if it suddenly develops, it may be a sign of one of many possible medical conditions including:

- Long-term lung disease or heart disease, such as bronchiectasis, chronic obstructive pulmonary disease, or endocarditis

- Inflammatory bowel disease, a long-term disease that causes inflammation of the lining of the gut

- Stomach cancer or bowel cancer

- Cirrhosis (scarring of the liver)

- Polycythemia, a condition where the blood is too thick

The easiest way to spot clubbed fingertips is to hold your fingers horizontally in front of you so you are looking at the nails side on. Normal nails should dip downwards towards the cuticle. With clubbed fingertips, this natural angle is gone and the nails are in line with the top of the fingers.

White Lines Running Across Nails

White spots or streaks are normal and nothing to worry about, but parallel white lines that extend all the way across the nails, known as Muehrcke's lines, are a sign of low levels of protein in the blood. This can be due to liver disease or malnutrition.

Dark Stripes Running Down The Nail

If you have dark skin, it's fairly common to find dark stripes running down your nails. This occurs in more than 77 percent of black people over the age of 20, and in most cases is perfectly normal.

However, it is not something to ignore: Dark stripes may sometimes be a form of skin cancer that affects the nail bed, called subungual melanoma. It's therefore important that your doctor checks it to rule out melanoma.

Generally, subungual melanoma only affects one nail. Also, it will cause the stripe to change in appearance (for example, it may become wider or darker over time) and the pigmentation may also affect the surrounding skin (the nail fold).

Red Or Brown Little Streaks Under The Nails

If you have what look like red or brown little streaks underneath the nails, it's likely these are splinter hemorrhages, or lines of blood caused by tiny damaged blood vessels.

Just a few splinters under one nail are nothing to worry about and most likely due to injury to the nail. However, if many nails are affected, these splinters may be a sign of an infection of the heart valves or another serious underlying disease.

A Destroyed Nail

The nail plate can be destroyed by:

- Injury, including nail biting

- Skin diseases such as psoriasis or lichen planus

- Overgrowth of the surrounding tissues, which is usually harmless (for example, due to a wart or verruca) but can sometimes be cancerous

If one of your nails becomes destroyed and you don't remember injuring it, it's important that you see your family doctor.

Painful, Red, And Swollen Nail Fold (Paronychia)

Paronychia is the name for inflammation of the nail folds, which are the skin and soft tissue that frame and support the nail.

This can be caused by infection, injury, irritation, or (rarely) a contact allergy or reaction to a drug. It's about three times more common in women than in men. Sometimes, there is an underlying skin condition such as eczema or psoriasis or another medical condition such as diabetes or HIV.

Paronychia can be acute, where it develops over a few hours, or chronic, where it lasts more than six weeks.

Acute infective paronychia usually starts after a minor injury to the nail fold, through nail biting, picking, or manicures, for example. The affected area is red, warm, tender, and swollen. After a while pus may be seen, which can track around the nail and even lift the nail off.

Acute paronychia is often caused by *Staphylococcus aureus* bacteria, although any number of germs can be involved. Treatment is with antibiotic creams and/or tablets. If there is a large amount of pus, it can help to have this surgically drained.

Sometimes, acute paronychia is caused by the cold sore virus, in which cased it is known as herpetic whitlow.

Acute paronychia can completely clear in a few days with treatment, but if it is not treated or does not respond to treatment, it can become chronic.

Chronic paronychia may start more gradually and be more difficult to get rid of. It is most common in people who often have their hands in water or chemicals, such as housewives, bartenders, cafeteria staff, or fishmongers.

It may start in one nail fold but can affect several fingers. The affected nail folds are swollen and may be red and sore from time to time, often after exposure to water. The nail plate gradually becomes thickened and ridged as it grows, and may become yellow or green and brittle.

The skin in chronic paronychia is often colonized by a mixture of yeasts and bacteria. This means these germs thrive on previously damaged skin, without necessarily starting the skin damage in the first place.

To settle chronic paronychia, both the skin damage and the colonization with germs needs to be addressed.

It can take months for chronic paronychia to clear, and after that up to a year for nails to grow back to normal. In the meantime, here's what you can do:

- Keep your hands dry and warm.
- Use waterproof gloves for any kind of wet work.
- Avoid biting or picking your nails.
- Avoid damaging your cuticles when manicuring your nails.
- Avoid exposure to chemicals, including nail polish, until the paronychia has settled.
- Apply an emollient hand cream frequently.
- Use an emollient hand cream instead of soap for washing your hands.

See your family doctor if the condition is severe. Depending on the type of paronychia, creams and/or tablets may be prescribed. Use these as directed.

You may be referred to a dermatologist for further investigation of the underlying skin disease or for contact allergy testing, and for treatment advice.

Part Six
Taking Care Of Your Skin, Hair, And Nails

Chapter 53

Skin And Hair Care

Beauty magazines show tons of beautiful girls and women in ads for hair and skin products. But, don't be fooled into thinking you need these products to look your best. Instead, try these time-tested beauty basics, which will keep you looking naturally beautiful.

Skin Care 101

1. Wash your face regularly using a mild cleanser and warm water. Be gentle—don't scrub hard! Avoid astringents, which can dry out and irritate skin.

2. Use only light, water-based moisturizers. Look for one that has SPF 15 or a higher number sunscreen.

3. For sensitive skin, try products that say "fragrance-free" or "without perfume."

4. If you're allowed to wear makeup, use only water-based products that say "noncomedogenic" or "nonacnegenic" on the label. Make sure to take off your makeup before going to bed.

5. To control acne, try over-the-counter products that you can buy without a doctor's order. These products come as gels, lotions, creams, and soaps. Your doctor can treat more serious acne problems.

6. Drink plenty of water.

7. Always wear "broad-spectrum" sunscreen, which protects against UVA and UVB rays. Wear sunscreen even on cloudy days. SPF alone does not protect against these two

About This Chapter: From "Teen Survival Guide: Hair And Skin Care," Office on Women's Health, February 12, 2008. Reviewed by David A. Cooke, MD, FACP, February 25, 2013.

types of harmful rays. Follow the directions on the bottle to put more on after a while. Wear lipscreen with at least SPF 15. And, your skin needs more than just sunscreen.

- Wear long-sleeve shirts, pants, and a hat.

- Stay in the shade.

- Stay out of the sun in the middle of the day, when rays are strongest.

Fun Quiz

The sun's UV rays are strongest between ___ a.m. and ___ p.m.

(Answer: 10 a.m. and 4 p.m.)

Hair Care 101

1. Wash your hair regularly, but only as often as you need to. Washing too often can strip away the natural oils that give hair shine and body.

2. If you see white flakes in your hair or on your shoulders, try a shampoo that treats dandruff. These shampoos are sold near other hair-care products.

3. Use shampoo, conditioners, and styling products that are right for your hair type.

4. Try different styles and looks. But beware of products that perm, relax, or color hair at home. They have chemicals that can damage your hair. Also, over-styling with hairdryers or curling and flattening irons can cause your hair to dry out or break.

5. Protect your hair and face from sun damage by wearing a hat or scarf that covers the back of your neck and face.

6. Protect your hair from chlorine (found in pool water) by wearing a swim cap or rinsing out your hair right after swimming. Soaking your hair with regular water before you put on your swim cap can also help.

Teen Tip

Wear wrap-around sunglasses that provide 100 percent UV ray protection. They look cool and keep your eyes safe.

Beauty Do's And Don'ts

- DO look your age. Heavy make-up hides your young, natural beauty—the beauty older women try so hard to get back!

- DON'T pop zits. This can cause infections and scars that are hard to get rid of.

- DO wear sunscreen. Protect your skin from the sun to help stop early wrinkles.

- DON'T be hard on yourself. Instead of thinking about what you don't like about your body, love the things that make you unique.

Does eating chocolate cause pimples?

No way—and neither do dirt, fried foods, or sexual activity. Changes in your skin during puberty trigger acne. Stress, your period, picking at or popping your pimples, scrubbing your skin too hard, getting too much sun and using oil-based lotions, makeup, or hair gels can cause breakouts to get worse.

Chapter 54

Sweating And Preventing Body Odor

Although it may seem like some strange disorder, it's actually perfectly normal to sweat. Sweating plays an important role in the body because it helps maintain body temperature by cooling us down. When we're hot and we sweat, that moisture evaporates and cools us off a bit. We don't just sweat when we are hot. It's also normal for people to sweat when they're nervous because emotions can affect the sweat glands.

Sweating is one part of puberty. When our bodies start to change, our roughly 3 million sweat glands become more active. This is especially true for glands in the armpits and groin and on the palms of the hands and soles of the feet. When the sweat comes in contact with bacteria on the skin, it can produce an odor, which may be stronger in some people than others.

So how to handle sweat? Take a bath or shower daily. If you're worried about smell, use a deodorant or a deodorant with antiperspirant (a deodorant masks odor, whereas an antiperspirant helps decrease sweating).

It can also help to wear clothes made of natural fibers, such as cotton or linen, especially in the summer heat. Pads called underarm shields or dress shields can also help absorb sweat and prevent embarrassing underarm stains. These pads attach to the armpit area inside a person's clothes where they absorb sweat. You can buy them in the lingerie departments of many department stores and at some specialized sports stores. Some teens also keep an extra shirt in their lockers so they can change at school.

About This Chapter: "Why Do I Sweat So Much?" September 2010, reprinted with permission from www .kidshealth.org. This information was provided by KidsHealth®, one of the largest resources online for medically reviewed health information written for parents, kids, and teens. For more articles like this, visit www.KidsHealth .org, or www.TeensHealth.org. Copyright © 1995-2012 The Nemours Foundation. All rights reserved.

If you still worry about your sweating, talk to a doctor. Occasionally sweating too much might be a sign of a medical problem. Stronger antiperspirants are now available with a doctor's prescription—your doctor may think a prescription-strength antiperspirant might help you.

Chapter 55

Sun Exposure

Tanning

To many people, summer means hanging out at the pool or the beach, soaking up rays in pursuit of a golden tan. But before you put on your bathing suit and head to the pool (or pay for a bed or booth in a tanning salon), there are a few things to think about when it comes to your skin and sun exposure.

How Tanning Happens

The sun's rays contain two types of ultraviolet radiation that reach your skin: UVA and UVB. UVB radiation burns the upper layers of skin (the epidermis), causing sunburns.

UVA radiation is what makes people tan. UVA rays penetrate to the lower layers of the epidermis, where they trigger cells called **melanocytes** (pronounced: mel-**an**-oh-sites) to produce **melanin**. Melanin is the brown pigment that causes tanning.

Melanin is the body's way of protecting skin from burning. Darker-skinned people tan more deeply than lighter-skinned people because their melanocytes produce more melanin. But just because a person doesn't burn does not mean that he or she is also protected against skin cancer and other problems.

Tanning Downsides

UVA rays may make you tan, but they can also cause serious damage. That's because UVA rays penetrate deeper into the skin than UVB rays. UVA rays can go all the way

About This Chapter: "Tanning," July 2012, reprinted with permission from www.kidshealth.org. This information was provided by KidsHealth®, one of the largest resources online for medically reviewed health information written for parents, kids, and teens. For more articles like this, visit www.KidsHealth.org, or www.TeensHealth .org. Copyright © 1995-2012 The Nemours Foundation. All rights reserved.

through the skin's protective epidermis to the dermis, where blood vessels and nerves are found.

Because of this, UVA rays may damage a person's immune system, making it harder to fight off diseases and leading to illnesses like melanoma, the most serious type of skin cancer. Melanoma can kill. If it's not found and treated, it can quickly spread from the skin to the body's other organs.

Skin cancer is epidemic in the United States, with more than 1 million new cases diagnosed every year. Although the numbers of new cases of many other types of cancer are falling or leveling off, the number of new melanoma cases is growing.

In the past, melanoma mostly affected people in their fifties or older, but today dermatologists see patients in their twenties and even late teens with this type of cancer. Experts believe this is partly due to an increase in the use of tanning beds and sun lamps, which have high levels of UVA rays. Getting a sunburn or intense sun exposure may also increase a person's chances of developing this deadly cancer.

Exposure to UVB rays also increases your risk of getting two other types of skin cancer: **basal** and **squamous cell carcinoma**.

The main treatment for skin cancers is cutting the tumors out. Since many basal or squamous cell carcinomas are on the face and neck, surgery to remove them can leave people with facial scars. The scars from surgery to remove melanomas can be anywhere on the body, and they're often large.

Cancer isn't the only problem associated with UV exposure. UVA damage is the main factor in premature skin aging. To get a good idea of how sunlight affects the skin, look at your parents' skin and see how different it is from yours. Much of that is due to sun exposure, not the age difference!

UV rays can also lead to another problem we associate with old people: the eye problem cataracts.

Sun Smarts

Staying out of the sun altogether may seem like the only logical answer. But who wants to live like a hermit? The key is to enjoy the sun sensibly, finding a balance between sun protection and those great summer activities like beach volleyball and swimming.

Vitamin D: "The Sunshine Vitamin"

Vitamin D helps the body absorb calcium and protects it in other ways. The body gets some of its vitamin D from food and some by making it from sunlight (specifically UVB rays.) You may have heard that you need to spend time in the sun to get enough of this vitamin. But that's not true. Plenty of UV rays still get through sunscreen to help the body get enough vitamin D.

Sunscreens block or change the effect of the sun's harmful rays. They're one of your best defenses against sun damage because they protect you without interfering with your comfort and activity levels.

The SPF number on a sunscreen shows the level of UVB protection it gives. **Sunscreens with a higher SPF number provide more defense against the sun's damaging UV rays.**

Here are some tips to enjoy the great outdoors while protecting your skin and eyes from sun damage:

- **Wear sunscreen with an SPF of at least 15 every day, even on cloudy days and when you don't plan on spending much time outdoors.** Wearing sunscreen every day is essential because as much as 80 percent of sun exposure is incidental—the type you get from walking your dog or eating lunch outside. If you don't want to wear a pure sunscreen, try a moisturizer with sunscreen in it, but make sure you put on enough.

- **Use a broad-spectrum sunscreen that blocks both UVA and UVB rays.** Ideally, it should also be hypoallergenic and noncomedogenic so it doesn't cause a rash or clog your pores.

- **Reapply sunscreen every 1½ to 2 hours**. If you're not sure you're putting on enough, switch to sunscreen with a higher SPF, like SPF 30. No matter what the SPF, the sun can break down the UVA ingredients in sunscreen. Even if you don't get a sunburn, UVA rays could still be doing unseen damage to your skin.

- **Reapply sunscreen after swimming or sweating.**

- **Take frequent breaks.** The sun's rays are strongest between 10 a.m. and 4 p.m. During those hours, take breaks to cool off indoors or in the shade for a while before heading out again.

- **Wear a hat with a brim and sunglasses that provide almost 100% protection against ultraviolet radiation.**

Other things to know when it comes to avoiding sun damage:

- You probably know that water is a major reflector of UV radiation—but so are sand, concrete, and even snow. Snow skiing and other winter activities carry significant risk of sunburn, so always apply sunblock before hitting the slopes.

- Certain medications, such as antibiotics used to treat acne and birth control pills, can increase your sun sensitivity (as well as your sensitivity to tanning beds). Ask your doctor whether your medications might have this effect and what you should do.

- Avoid tanning "accelerators" or tanning pills that claim to speed up the body's production of melanin or darken the skin. There's no proof that they work and they aren't approved by government agencies for tanning purposes.

Trauma-Free Tans

Even when you're serious about protecting your skin, you may sometimes want the glow of a tan. Luckily, many products on the market—but not sun lamps or tanning beds—will let you tan safely and sun-free.

One safe way to go bronze is with sunless self-tanners. These "tans in a bottle" contain dihydroxyacetone (DHA), which gradually stains the dead cells in your skin's outer layer. The "tan" lasts until these skin cells slough off, so exfoliating or vigorously washing will make the color fade faster. Typically, self-tanners last from several days to a week.

You may have to try a few brands of self-tanner to find one that looks best with your skin tone. For a subtle, goof-proof glow, try moisturizers that contain a modest amount of fake tanner, letting you gradually build up a little color without blotches and staining—or the smell that some people dislike. All of these options are cheap, too, usually around $10.

Ask a friend to help you apply self-tanner to spots you can't reach, like your back. And be sure to wash your hands as soon as you finish applying the tanner. Areas of your body that don't normally tan (like the palms of your hands or soles of the feet) just look dirty if you leave tanner on them.

With self-tanners, you get better results if you exfoliate your skin with a scrub brush or loofah before the tanner is applied. This evens your skin tone and removes dead skin cells.

If you use a sunless tanner, you'll need to wear plenty of sunscreen when you go outdoors to protect you from the sun's rays. Self-tanners don't generate melanin production, so they won't protect you against sunburn (and some scientists believe they might even make skin more susceptible to sun damage).

If you're thinking about using a sunless tanner, **it's a good idea to avoid airbrush or spray-on tans.** The Food and Drug Administration (FDA) hasn't approved DHA for use internally or on mucous membranes (like the lips). Spray tans may have unknown health risks because people can breathe in the spray, or the tanner may end up on their lips or eye area.

Tans Weren't Always the Rage

Being as pale as possible was once desirable in some countries because a tan was the sign of manual labor. The wealthy could afford to have other people do that work for them, so the paler people were, the richer they seemed. Then in the 1920s designer Coco Chanel returned from a vacation to the Riviera with a deep tan and suddenly tans were the badges of the rich.

Chapter 56

Indoor Tanning

Using a tanning bed, booth, or sunlamp to get tan is called "indoor tanning." Indoor tanning has been linked with skin cancers including melanoma (the deadliest type of skin cancer), squamous cell carcinoma, and cancers of the eye (ocular melanoma).

Dangers Of Indoor Tanning

Indoor tanning exposes users to both UV-A and UV-B rays, which damage the skin and can lead to cancer. Using a tanning bed is particularly dangerous for younger users; people who begin tanning younger than age 35 have a 75 percent higher risk of melanoma. Using tanning beds also increases the risk of wrinkles and eye damage, and changes skin texture.

Myths About Indoor Tanning

"Tanning indoors is safer than tanning in the sun."

Indoor tanning and tanning outside are both dangerous. Although tanning beds operate on a timer, the exposure to ultraviolet (UV) rays can vary based on the age and type of light bulbs. You can still get a burn from tanning indoors, and even a tan indicates damage to your skin.

"I can use a tanning bed to get a base tan, which will protect me from getting a sunburn."

A tan is a response to injury: Skin cells respond to damage from UV rays by producing more pigment. The best way to protect your skin from the sun is by using these tips for skin cancer prevention:

About This Chapter: From "Indoor Tanning," Centers for Disease Control and Prevention (www.cdc.gov), July 16, 2012.

Citing Risks Of Cancer, States Seek To Limit Teen Tanning

Legislators and cancer researchers are trying to turn out the lights on indoor tanning for teens. Lawmakers in 12 states are currently debating bills restricting tanning bed use for anyone under age 18, with some states allowing parental consent and other imposing an outright ban, according to analysis from the National Conference of State Legislatures.

Currently, 27 states have laws requiring parental consent for teen tanning under ages 17 and 18. Minnesota and Connecticut require parental consent for teens under16, and Virginia for teens under 15.

Legislators are responding to new research that directly links indoor tanning to skin cancer. Tanning booths deliver 10 to 15 times the UV radiation of natural sunlight, boosting the user's risk of developing deadly melanoma by at least 75 percent, according to the Skin Cancer Foundation. Teenage girls, one of the largest demographics of tanners, are more susceptible to melanoma than other groups, according to the National Cancer Institute. Its research found that melanoma is the second most common form of cancer for young people 15–29 years old.

These bans have not gone over well with tanning salon owners and the Indoor Tanning Association, a Washington, D.C.-based advocacy group that lobbies on behalf of the tanning industry. But interest in the bans generally fades when concerned tanners speak to state lawmakers, says Executive Director John Overstreet. He points to efforts in Florida, West Virginia, and Washington this year [in 2012] where bans were debated, but ultimately failed.

"Thus far," Overstreet says, "things are progressing OK this year. The secret in this is that the people in the state have to speak up."

In Utah, the state with the highest rate of melanoma skin cancer in the nation, according to the Centers for Disease Control, lawmakers earlier this month approved a bill that will require parents to accompany their children under 18 to any tanning salon, and require the salon to give the parent a written notice of the risks associated with indoor tanning.

"Parents have a right to know when their children are taking on a known carcinogen," said Rep. Brad Wilson, House sponsor of the tanning restrictions, in an interview with the *Deseret News*. "This is something that is so risky that we ought to have a parent know every time a child goes in to do this…I know this bill will save lives."

The Food and Drug Administration, which regulates tanning beds, has not taken a formal position on the issue of teen tanning, but the agency is considering modifying regulations for tanning beds to reduce the amount of UV exposures.

Source: "Citing Risks of Cancer, States Seek to Limit Teen Tanning," March 19, 2012. Reprinted from *Stateline*, www.pew-center-states.com. *Stateline* is a nonpartisan, nonprofit news service of the Pew Center on the States that provides daily reporting and analysis on trends in state policy. © 2012. All rights reserved. Author: Maggie Clark, *Stateline* staff writer.

What's It Mean?

Indoor Tanning: Using a tanning bed, booth, or sunlamp to get a tan.

Melanoma: Deadliest type of skin cancer.

Ocular Melanoma: Cancers of the eye.

Squamous Cell Carcinoma: A type of skin cancer linked to indoor tanning.

Sun Protective Factor (SPF): The level of skin protection found in sunscreen.

Ultraviolet (UV) Rays: Radiation from the sun or indoor tanning.

—LE

- Seek shade, especially during midday hours.

- Wear clothing to protect exposed skin.

- Wear a hat with a wide brim to shade the face, head, ears, and neck.

- Wear sunglasses that wrap around and block as close to 100% of both UVA and UVB rays as possible.

- Use sunscreen with sun protective factor (SPF) 15 or higher, and both UVA and UVB protection.

- Avoid indoor tanning.

"Indoor tanning is a safe way to get vitamin D, which prevents many health problems."

Vitamin D is important for bone health, but studies showing links between vitamin D and other health conditions are inconsistent. Although it is important to get enough vitamin D, the safest way is through diet or supplements. Tanning harms your skin, and the amount of time spent tanning to get enough vitamin D varies from person to person.

Statistics

According to the 2011 Youth Risk Behavior Surveillance System, the following proportions of youth report indoor tanning:

- 13 percent of all high school students

- 21 percent of high school girls

- 32 percent of girls in the 12th grade

- 29 percent of white high school girls

According to the 2010 National Health Interview Survey, indoor tanners tended to be young, non-Hispanic white women.

- Thirty-two percent of non-Hispanic white women aged 18–21 years reported indoor tanning. Those who reported indoor tanning device use reported an average of 28 sessions in the past year.

- Among non-Hispanic white adults who used an indoor tanning device in the past year, 58 percent of women and 40 percent of men used one 10 times or more in the past year.

- Non-Hispanic white women between the ages of 18 and 21 years residing in the Midwest (44 percent) and non-Hispanic white women between the ages of 22 and 25 old in the South (36 percent) were most likely to use indoor tanning devices.

Indoor Tanning Policies

Indoor tanning is restricted in some areas, especially for minors.

United States

- California and Vermont have banned the use of tanning beds by minors.

- Some local jurisdictions also have banned the use of tanning beds by minors.

International

- Brazil and one state in Australia (New South Wales) have banned the use of tanning beds.

- The United Kingdom, Germany, Scotland, France, several Australian states, and several Canadian provinces have banned indoor tanning for people younger than age 18.

Chapter 57

Tanning Alternatives

Despite the fact that young adults are generally in constant communication via social media and texting, a new survey finds many in this age group are not getting the message that there is no such thing as a safe tan.

The survey, conducted by the American Academy of Dermatology (Academy), determined that young adults are not aware of the danger of tanning beds and how to properly protect their skin from sun damage.

Survey Statistics

- Nearly one-half (45 percent) of young adult respondents agreed with the statement "I prefer to enjoy sunshine and not worry about what I should do to protect myself from it," compared with one-third of overall respondents.

- Nearly one-quarter (24 percent) of young adults were either unaware or unsure that tanning beds are not safer than the sun.

- Only 35 percent of young respondents 18 to 29 knew that a base tan is not a healthy way to protect the skin from sun damage.

- Three in 10 (31 percent) of young adults were either unsure or unaware that sun exposure can cause wrinkles.

About This Chapter: Text in this chapter is from "Dermatologists Give Young Adults Something To Tweet About: Tanning Is Out," May 4, 2012. Reprinted with permission from the American Academy of Dermatology (www.aad.org), © 2012. All rights reserved.

"It's troubling that so many young adults do not fully understand the consequences of tanning—whether from tanning beds or natural sunlight—particularly in light of the trend of more young people developing skin cancer," said board-certified dermatologist Amanda Friedrichs, MD, FAAD. "Our survey confirmed that age was highly associated with the use of tanning beds, as respondents 18 to 29 years old were much more likely than those over 30 to report using a tanning bed."

For young adults who insist on looking tan, Dr. Friedrichs recommends using a self-tanner rather than exposing one's skin to harmful ultraviolet radiation. In the past, self-tanners had a reputation of turning skin orange, streaking, and splotching, but Dr. Friedrichs offered these basic tips for applying a self-tanner to get even coverage and longer-lasting results:

- **Exfoliate.** Prior to using a self-tanner, use a washcloth to exfoliate the skin. Using an exfoliating product will also help remove the dead skin cells. Spend a little more time exfoliating where the skin is thickest, such as the ankles, knees, and elbows.

- **Dry the skin.** Drying your skin before you apply a self-tanner helps it go on evenly.

- **Apply in sections.** Apply the self-tanner in sections, such as the arms, legs, and torso. Massage the self-tanner into the skin with a uniform circular motion. Lightly extend the tanner from the wrists to the hands and from the ankles to the feet, taking care not to treat the entire hands and feet, such as the palms and soles. Wash and dry your hands after applying self-tanner to each body part to avoid tanning your palms.

- **Dilute tanner on joints.** Dilute the self-tanner on the knees, ankles, and elbows, since these areas tend to absorb more self-tanner than the rest of the skin. To dilute, lightly rub these areas with a damp towel or apply a lotion.

- **Allow time to dry.** Wait at least 10 minutes before getting dressed. It's best to wear loose clothing and try to avoid sweating for the next three hours.

"Self-tanning products will make you look tan, but it's important to remember that you still need a broad-spectrum sunscreen with an SPF of 30 or higher while you are outdoors," said Dr. Friedrichs. "While self-tanners are a safe alternative to tanning, people need to be vigilant about protecting their skin from sun exposure and avoid indoor tanning to reduce their risk of skin cancer to avoid premature aging of the skin."

Dr. Friedrichs' tips are demonstrated in "Self-Tanner: How To Apply," a video posted to the Academy website and the Academy's YouTube channel. This video is first in the Dermatology A to Z video series, which offers relatable videos that demonstrate tips people can use to properly care for their skin, hair, and nails. A new video in the series will be posted to the Academy website and the YouTube channel each month, beginning in May 2012.

Sunless Tanners And Bronzers

What are "sunless tanners?"

Neither the laws nor the regulations enforced by U.S. Food and Drug Administration (FDA) define the term "sunless tanner." It typically refers to products that provide a tanned appearance without exposure to the sun or other sources of ultraviolet radiation. One commonly used ingredient in these products is dihydroxyacetone (DHA), a color additive that darkens the skin by reacting with amino acids in the skin's surface.

What are "bronzers?"

The term "bronzer" is not defined in either the laws or the regulations enforced by FDA. It is often used to describe a variety of products intended to achieve a temporary tanned appearance. For example, among the products marketed as bronzers are tinted moisturizers and brush-on powders. These produce a temporary effect, similar to other types of makeup, and wash off over time. Some products are marketed with other ingredients in addition to DHA in order to provide a tanned appearance.

What does this mean for DHA spray "tanning" booths?

The use of DHA in "tanning" booths as an all-over spray has not been approved by the FDA, since safety data to support this use has not been submitted to the Agency for review and evaluation. When using DHA-containing products as an all-over spray or mist in a commercial spray "tanning" booth, it may be difficult to avoid exposure in a manner for which DHA is not approved, including the area of the eyes, lips, or mucous membrane, or even internally.

Consumers should request measures to protect their eyes and mucous membranes and prevent inhalation.

What about sunless tanning products sold in retail stores, such as creams and lotions?

DHA is approved for external application to the human body, which is the way these products are intended to be used. Consumers can easily avoid inhaling them or applying them to the area of the eye or mucous membrane.

Do sunless tanners and bronzers provide protection from the sun?

Sunless tanners and bronzers may or may not provide protection from the sun. Only those sunless tanners that contain sunscreen ingredients and are labeled with sun protection factor ("SPF") numbers may provide protection. Consumers are advised to read the labeling carefully to determine whether or not these products provide protection from the sun.

Source: Excerpted from "Sunless Tanners And Bronzers," U.S. Food and Drug Administration (www.fda.gov), December 7, 2012.

Skin Cancer Facts

- Melanoma is the most common form of skin cancer for young adults 25 to 29 years old, and the second-most-common for teens and young adults 15 to 29 years old.

- Melanoma is increasing faster in females 15 to 29 years old than males in the same age group.

- It is estimated that there will be about 131,810 new cases of melanoma in 2012—55,560 noninvasive (*in situ*) and 76,250 invasive (44,250 men and 32,000 women).

- Exposure to tanning beds increases the risk of melanoma, especially in women aged 45 years or younger.

In an effort to increase the public's awareness of skin cancer and motivate people to change their behavior to prevent and detect skin cancer, the Academy launched the new SPOT Skin Cancer™ public awareness campaign in May 2012. The campaign's simple tagline—"Prevent. Detect. Live."—focuses on the positive actions people can take to protect themselves from skin cancer, including seeing a board-certified dermatologist when appropriate.

Chapter 58

Tattoos And Tattoo Removal

Tattoo Inks Pose Health Risks

Tempted to get a tattoo? Today, people from all walks of life have tattoos, which might lead you to believe that tattoos are completely safe.

But there are health risks that can result in the need for medical care. The Food and Drug Administration (FDA) is particularly concerned about a family of bacteria called nontuberculous mycobacteria (NTM) that has been found in a recent outbreak of illnesses linked to contaminated tattoo inks.

M. chelonae, one of several disease-causing NTM species, can cause lung disease, joint infection, eye problems, and other organ infections. These infections can be difficult to diagnose and can require treatment lasting six months or more.

Some of these contaminated inks have caused serious infections in at least four states in late 2011 and early 2012. FDA is reaching out to tattoo artists, ink and pigment manufacturers, public health officials, health care professionals, and consumers to warn them of the potential for infection.

FDA also warns that tattoo inks, and the pigments used to color them, can become contaminated by other bacteria, mold, and fungi. To raise awareness and make diagnoses more accurate, FDA strongly encourages reporting of tattoo-associated complications to its MedWatch program, says Linda Katz, M.D., M.P.H., director of FDA's Office of Cosmetics and Colors.

About This Chapter: This chapter begins with information excerpted from "Tattoo Inks Pose Health Risks," U.S. Food and Drug Administration (www.fda.gov), August 22, 2012. Additional information from Cleveland Clinic is cited separately within the chapter.

Getting the word out to tattoo artists is particularly critical. Even when they diligently follow hygienic practices, they may not know that an ink itself may be contaminated. Contamination is not always visible in the inks, Katz says.

FDA's goal is to encourage these artists to take certain precautions in their practice and to urge potentially infected clients to seek medical care. "Reporting an infection to FDA and the artist is important. Once the problem is reported, FDA can investigate, and the artist can take steps to prevent others from being infected," says epidemiologist Katherine Hollinger, D.V.M., M.P.H., from the Office of Cosmetics and Colors.

Strategies For Controlling Risks Of Infection

Tattoo artists can minimize the risk of infection by using inks that have been formulated or processed to ensure they are free from disease-causing bacteria, and avoiding the use of non-sterile water to dilute the inks or wash the skin. Non-sterile water includes tap, bottled, filtered, or distilled water.

Consumers should know that the ointments often provided by tattoo parlors are not effective against these infections. NTM infections may look similar to allergic reactions, which means they might be easily misdiagnosed and treated ineffectively.

Once an infection is diagnosed, health care providers will prescribe appropriate antibiotic treatment, according to Katz. Such treatment might have uncomfortable side effects, such as nausea or gastrointestinal problems. However, without prompt and proper treatment, an infection could spread beyond the tattoo or become complicated by a secondary infection.

If you suspect you may have a tattoo-related infection, FDA recommends the following steps:

- Contact your health care professional if you see a red rash with swelling, possibly accompanied by itching or pain in the tattooed area, usually appearing two to three weeks after tattooing.

- Report the problem to the tattoo artist.

- Report the problem to MedWatch, on the web or at 800-332-1088; or contact FDA's consumer complaint coordinator in your area.

Why Tattoo Inks Go Bad

Inks and pigments can be contaminated in these ways:

- Use of contaminated ingredients to make inks

- Use of manufacturing processes that introduce contaminants or allow contaminants to survive

- Use of unhygienic practices that contaminate ink bottles or mixing with contaminated colors

- Use of non-sterile water to dilute the inks

- Using tattoo inks past their expiration date

Tattoo Removal

Laser Therapy Now Light Years Ahead

In the past, tattoos were surgically shaved, scraped or frozen off, or peeled away with chemicals. "Frequently, this left an undesirable scar," notes Dr. Allison Vidimos, Chairman of Dermatology and Vice Chairman of the Dermatologic & Plastic Surgery Institute at the Cleveland Clinic.

Carbon dioxide lasers were the first lasers ever used to remove both tattoos and the scars from removal attempts. In the 1980s, "Q-switched" lasers emerged, offering better results. Their tiny pulses of high-powered energy remove or fade most colors, with little risk of skin damage. A series of laser treatments, four to eight weeks apart, is usually required.

12 Tips To Consider Before Scheduling Tattoo Removal

1. Some tattoos fade only partially after laser treatments.

2. Older tattoos fade more easily than newer ones.

3. Fading is generally slower for tattoos located further down the arm or leg.

4. Amateur tattoos are usually easier to remove than professional tattoos.

5. No single laser can remove all tattoo colors. Different dyes respond to different light wavelengths.

6. Black and dark green are the easiest colors to remove; yellow, purple, turquoise, and fluorescent dyes are hardest.

7. Tattooing itself may scar or change skin texture, an effect often hidden by the dyes. If laser removal uncovers skin changes, you may be left with what looks like a "ghost" of your old tattoo.

8. Laser treatments may darken or lighten skin pigment over and around the tattoo.

9. Apply sunscreen before and after laser tattoo removal to minimize changes in your skin pigment. For the same reason, wait for your tan to fade before having a tattoo removed.

10. Certain cosmetic tattoos, such as red, white, and flesh-colored lip liners, may darken immediately with laser therapy. (This effect can usually be corrected with further treatment.)

11. If immediate skin darkening is a concern, the laser should be tested on a small spot first.

12. If you experienced an allergic reaction when getting your tattoo—intense itching and swelling of dyed area(s)—tell your doctor. Using a "Q-switched" laser to remove the tattoo can trigger a more serious allergic reaction.

Finally, before getting more body art, remember that it is meant to be permanent. "Make sure the tattoo you get is one you won't mind having later in life," says Dr. Vidimos.

Chapter 59

Piercing

Piercing And Teens

Piercing is popular among today's teens. Most parents with eventually hear the question: "Mom/Dad, can I get my [body part] pierced?"

Here is some information you need to know.

How Is It Done?

A hollow needle is passed through the body part, and jewelry is inserted into the hole. A piercing gun should not be used because it crushes the tissues that are pierced and it cannot be properly sterilized.

How Do The Holes Heal?

Skin heals after piercing by forming a layer of cells called epithelial cells along the inside of the piercing. This protects the body from the foreign object. The epithelial cells form a tube-like layer of skin along the inside of the piercing. The process takes at least six to eight weeks, although most body piercings require at least six months to a year before the jewelry can be removed for any length of time without the risk of the hole closing.

After the epithelial layer has formed, the piercing may constrict around the jewelry. The epithelial layer can be easily torn or dislodged, so do not force the jewelry to rotate without first applying warm water. Once the epithelial cell layer forms, it must toughen and strengthen for up to a year before the piercing will become more flexible and relaxed around the jewelry.

About This Chapter: "Piercing And Teens," reprinted with permission from the Palo Alto Medical Foundation Teen Health website, http://www.pamf.org/teen. © 2012 Palo Alto Medical Foundation. All rights reserved. Author: PAMF Senior Research Associate Nancy Brown, Ph.D., M.A., Ed.S.

Caring For The Piercing Site

- First, make sure that your piercing is done with a sterile object (single use), and that jewelry inserted in the new piercing site is also sterile. This prevents bacteria and foreign objects from entering the body.

- All new piercing produces a sticky white or off-white discharge that dries into a crusty formation around the opening of the piercing and on the jewelry. The area around the new piercing should be kept clean.

- Do not touch the new piercing (unless cleaning it). Wash your hands with antibacterial soap before cleaning the piercing.

- Sea salt-water soaks are good to loosen up crusty formations. You can make salt water by adding ¼ teaspoon of salt to 12 ounces of clean water.

- For piercing in your ear or around your face, avoid make-up and powders in that area during the healing process. Cover the pierced area with a tissue when applying hair spray.

- For body piercing, do not wear tight clothes.

- For navel piercing, do not wear large belts, stockings, or body suits, and do not sleep on your stomach. Good air circulation is important for healing.

- Be careful where you swim. Avoid public pools and hot tubs until the piercing has healed.

Signs Of Infection

See your health care provider if you experience any of the following:

- Pain that does not go away within a day or two

- Increased pain, unusual pain or swelling in the piercing site

- If the area feels hot to the touch

- If you see red lines starting from piercing

- If you see oozing, bleeding, pus

Do not remove your jewelry. If the jewelry is removed, the openings of the piercing may close and trap the infection, which can create an abscess (a pus-filled, painful area).

Oral Piercing And Dental Health

No matter where you get a piercing, you could have an infection or sensitivity. Piercings in the mouth have some specific additional risks, according to the American Dental Association.

Metal jewelry in the mouth can cause irritation to the soft tissue in the mouth, and it can cause the gums to recede due to constant irritation. Constant contact of the jewelry against the teeth can cause chipping and cracking of the teeth, and jewelry that comes unfastened can be a choking hazard.

Picking A Studio: Where To Get It Done?

If you say yes to the piercing, consider accompanying your teen to the piercing studio. Have your teen research local piercing studios and select one based on these criteria:

- Is the shop clean, well lit, and licensed by the county?

- Does the studio use an autoclave to sterilize equipment?

- Are needles used only once and thrown away?

- Is a consent form and photo ID required?

- Does the piercer use gloves and wash his or her hands thoroughly between customers?

Then, make an appointment and go together. You will both need a photo ID. You can ask the piercer to discuss the health issues before the piercing and the aftercare guidelines after the piercing.

Chapter 60

Hair Loss: Alopecia Areata

Questions And Answers About Alopecia Areata

This chapter contains general information about alopecia areata (al-oh-PEE-shah ar-ee-AH-tah). It describes what alopecia areata is, its causes, and treatment options.

If you have further questions after reading this chapter, you may wish to discuss them with your doctor.

Alopecia areata is just one cause of alopecia, or hair loss.

What is alopecia areata?

Alopecia areata is considered an autoimmune disease, in which the immune system, which is designed to protect the body from foreign invaders such as viruses and bacteria, mistakenly attacks the hair follicles, the structures from which hairs grow. This can lead to hair loss on the scalp and elsewhere.

In most cases, hair falls out in small, round patches about the size of a quarter. In many cases, the disease does not extend beyond a few bare patches. In some people, hair loss is more extensive. Although uncommon, the disease can progress to cause total loss of hair on the scalp (referred to as alopecia areata totalis) or complete loss of hair on the scalp, face, and body (alopecia areata universalis).

About This Chapter: From "Alopecia Areata," National Institute of Arthritis and Musculoskeletal and Skin Diseases (www.niams.nih.gov), January 2012.

What causes it?

In alopecia areata, immune system cells called white blood cells attack the rapidly growing cells in the hair follicles.

The affected hair follicles become small and drastically slow down hair production. Fortunately, the stem cells that continuously supply the follicle with new cells do not seem to be targeted. So the follicle always has the potential to regrow hair.

Scientists do not know exactly why the hair follicles undergo these changes, but they suspect that a combination of genes may predispose some people to the disease. In those who are genetically predisposed, some type of trigger—perhaps a virus or something in the person's environment—brings on the attack against the hair follicles.

Who is most likely to get it?

Alopecia areata affects nearly 2 percent of Americans of both sexes and of all ages and ethnic backgrounds. It often begins in childhood.

If you have a close family member with the disease, your risk of developing it is slightly increased. If your family member lost his or her first patch of hair before age 30, the risk to other family members is greater. Overall, one in five people with the disease has a family member who has it as well.

Is my hair loss a symptom of a serious disease?

Alopecia areata is not a life-threatening disease. It does not cause any physical pain, and people with the condition are generally healthy otherwise. But for most people, a disease that unpredictably affects their appearance the way alopecia areata does is a serious matter.

The effects of alopecia areata are primarily socially and emotionally disturbing. In alopecia universalis, however, loss of eyelashes and eyebrows and hair in the nose and ears can make the person more vulnerable to dust, germs, and foreign particles entering the eyes, nose, and ears.

Hair Loss And Steroid Abuse

Steroids—the kind that some athletes abuse—affect your appearance. In both sexes, steroids can cause male-pattern baldness, cysts, acne, and oily hair and skin. For girls: growth of facial hair.

Source: "Tips for Teens: The Truth About Steroids," U.S. Substance Abuse and Mental Health Services Administration (www.samhsa.gov), 2008. Reviewed by David A. Cooke, MD, FACP, March 2013.

Alopecia areata often occurs in people whose family members have other autoimmune diseases, such as type 1 diabetes, rheumatoid arthritis, thyroid disease, systemic lupus erythematosus, pernicious anemia, or Addison's disease. People who have alopecia areata do not usually have other autoimmune diseases, but they do have a higher occurrence of thyroid disease, atopic eczema, nasal allergies, and asthma.

Will my hair ever grow back?

There is every chance that your hair will regrow with or without treatment, but it may also fall out again. No one can predict when it might regrow or fall out. The course of the disease varies from person to person. Some people lose just a few patches of hair, then the hair regrows, and the condition never recurs. Other people continue to lose and regrow hair for many years. A few lose all the hair on the scalp; some lose all the hair on the scalp, face, and body. Even in those who lose all their hair, the possibility for full regrowth remains.

In some, the initial hair regrowth is white, with a gradual return of the original hair color. In most, the regrown hair is ultimately the same color and texture as the original hair.

What can I expect next?

The course of alopecia areata is highly unpredictable, and the uncertainty of what will happen next is probably the most difficult and frustrating aspect of the disease. You may continue to lose hair, or your hair loss may stop. The hair you have lost may or may not grow back, and you may or may not continue to develop new bare patches.

How is it treated?

Although there is neither a cure for alopecia areata nor drugs approved for its treatment, some people find that medications approved for other purposes can help hair grow back, at least temporarily. The following are some treatments for alopecia areata. Keep in mind that although these treatments may promote hair growth, none of them prevent new patches or actually cure the underlying disease. Consult your health care professional about the best option for you. A combination of treatments may work best. Ask how long the treatment may last, how long it will take before you see results, and about the possible side effects.

- **Corticosteroids:** Corticosteroids are powerful anti-inflammatory drugs similar to a hormone called cortisol, which is produced in the body. Because these drugs suppress the immune system if given orally, they are often used in the treatment of various autoimmune diseases, including alopecia areata. Corticosteroids may be administered in three ways for alopecia areata:

- **Local Injections:** Injections of steroids directly into hairless patches on the scalp, and sometimes the brow and beard areas, are effective in increasing hair growth in most people, and are the most common treatment in adults in the United States. Injections deliver small amounts of cortisone to affected areas, avoiding the more serious side effects encountered with long-term oral use. Side effects may include transient pain, as well as temporary depressions in the skin that usually fill in by themselves.

- **Oral Corticosteroids:** Corticosteroids taken by mouth are a mainstay of treatment for many autoimmune diseases and may be used in extensive alopecia areata. But because of the risk of side effects of oral corticosteroids, such as hypertension, weight gain, osteoporosis, and cataracts, they are used only occasionally for alopecia areata and for short periods of time.

- **Topical Ointments:** Ointments or creams containing steroids rubbed directly onto the affected area are less traumatic than injections and, therefore, are sometimes preferred for children. However, corticosteroid ointments and creams alone are less effective than injections.

- **Minoxidil (5%):** Topical minoxidil solution promotes hair growth in several conditions in which the hair follicle is small and not growing to its full potential. Minoxidil is approved by the U.S. Food and Drug Administration (FDA) for treating male and female pattern hair loss. It may also be useful in promoting hair growth in alopecia areata. The topical solution, applied twice daily, has been shown to promote hair growth in both adults and children, and may be used on the scalp, eyebrow, and beard areas.

- **Anthralin:** Anthralin, a synthetic tar-like substance that alters immune function in the affected skin, is an approved treatment for psoriasis. Anthralin is also commonly used to treat alopecia areata. It is applied topically.

- **Topical Sensitizers:** Topical sensitizers are medications that, when applied to the scalp, provoke an allergic reaction that leads to itching, scaling, and eventually hair growth. Two topical sensitizers are used in alopecia areata: squaric acid dibutyl ester (SADBE) and diphenylcyclopropenone (DPCP). They should be administered by doctors familiar with these products.

- **Photochemotherapy:** In photochemotherapy, a treatment used most commonly for psoriasis, a person is given a light-sensitive drug called a psoralen either orally or topically and then exposed to an ultraviolet light source. This combined treatment is called PUVA. Patients must go to a treatment center where the equipment is available at least two to three times per week. If used for long periods, the treatment may increase the risk of developing skin cancer.

- **Alternative Therapies:** When drug treatments fail to bring sufficient hair regrowth, some people turn to alternative therapies. Alternatives purported to help alopecia areata include acupuncture, aromatherapy, evening primrose oil, zinc and vitamin supplements, and Chinese herbs. Most alternative therapies are not backed by clinical trials, and because hair can regrow spontaneously in alopecia areata, it is difficult to evaluate the effectiveness of these alternatives. Furthermore, just because these therapies are natural does not mean that they are safe. As with any therapy, it is best to discuss these treatments with your doctor before you try them.

In addition to treatments to help hair grow, there are measures that can be taken to minimize the effects of excessive sun exposure or discomforts of lost hair.

- Sunscreens are important for the scalp, face, and all exposed areas.

- Eyeglasses (or sunglasses) protect the eyes from excessive sun and from dust and debris when eyebrows or eyelashes are missing.

- Wigs, caps, or scarves protect the scalp from the sun and keep the head warm.

- An ointment applied inside the nostrils keeps them moisturized and helps to protect against organisms invading the nose when nostril hair is missing.

How will alopecia areata affect my life?

This is a common question, particularly for children, teens, and young adults who are beginning to form lifelong goals and who may live with the effects of alopecia areata for many years. The comforting news is that alopecia areata is not a painful disease and does not make people feel sick physically. It is not contagious, and people who have the disease are generally healthy otherwise. It does not reduce life expectancy and it should not interfere with going to school, playing sports and exercising, pursuing any career, working, marrying, and raising a family.

The emotional aspects of living with hair loss, however, can be challenging. Many people cope by learning as much as they can about the disease, speaking with others who are facing the same problem, and, if necessary, seeking counseling to help build a positive self-image.

How can I cope with the effects of this disease?

Living with hair loss can be difficult, especially in a culture that views hair as a sign of youth and good health. Even so, most people with alopecia areata are well-adjusted, contented people living full lives.

The key to coping is valuing yourself for who you are, not for how much hair you have or don't have. Many people learning to cope with alopecia areata find it helpful to talk with other people who are dealing with the same problems. Nearly 2 percent of Americans have this disease at some point in their lives, so you are not alone. If you would like to be in touch with others with the disease, the National Alopecia Areata Foundation (NAAF) can help through its pen pal program, message boards, annual conference, and support groups that meet in various locations nationwide.

Another way to cope with the disease is to minimize its effects on your appearance. If you have extensive hair loss, a wig or hairpiece can look natural and stylish. For small patches of hair loss, a hair-colored powder, cream, or crayon applied to the scalp can make hair loss less obvious by eliminating the contrast between the hair and the scalp. Skillfully applied eyebrow pencil can mask missing eyebrows.

Children with alopecia areata may prefer to wear bandanas or caps. There are many styles available to suit a child's interest and mood. It is often helpful if a parent informs teachers, coaches, and others that the child has alopecia areata, that it is not contagious, and that the child is healthy.

For women, attractive scarves can hide patchy hair loss, and proper makeup can camouflage the effects of lost facial hair. If you would like to learn more about camouflaging the cosmetic aspects of alopecia areata, ask your doctor or members of your local support group to recommend a cosmetologist who specializes in working with people whose appearance is affected by medical conditions.

Chapter 61

Care For Healthy And Damaged Hair

While the latest hairstyles and hair colors may look great, dermatologists warn that many women are subjecting their hair to harsh chemicals and heated styling devices that, in turn, can damage the hair. Over time, lustrous hair can look lackluster, become brittle and require a complete hair care overhaul to improve hair health and appearance.

Speaking in 2011 at the 69th Annual Meeting of the American Academy of Dermatology (Academy), dermatologist Zoe D. Draelos, MD, FAAD, consulting professor at Duke University School of Medicine, Durham, N.C., discussed the most common sources of hair damage and tips to reverse damage and maintain healthy, lustrous hair.

"One of the most common misconceptions about hair is that it is alive, when in fact hair is nonliving and does not heal itself once it is injured," said Dr. Draelos. "For this reason, once the hair is damaged it cannot heal itself except through new hair growth at the scalp. Women need to understand that the very things that they do to hair to make it appear beautiful, such as using hair dyes, perms, and products that straighten the hair, will eventually end up damaging the hair's structure and ultimately affect its appearance."

Getting To The Root Of Chemical Hair Damage

When hair is damaged, the protective lipid layer of fat on the outside of the cuticle—responsible for making the hair shiny—is removed. Chemical damage is one of the most common culprits of hair damage, as processed hair loses its natural moisturizers. The result is dried-out, frizzy hair that does not hold its style and accounts for the hair's dull appearance.

About This Chapter: From "Going To Great Lengths For Beautiful Hair: Dermatologists Share Hair Care Tips For Healthy And Damaged Hair," February 4, 2011. Reprinted with permission from the American Academy of Dermatology (www.aad.org), © 2011. All rights reserved.

"Many products have been developed to counter the effects of over-processed hair, and regular moisturizing is a must for women with visible signs of hair damage," said Dr. Draelos.

Dr. Draelos offered this tips to combat chemical damage:

- Use conditioning shampoos and conditioners regularly to improve the appearance of frizzy hair. Two-in-one shampoos that remove oil from the scalp, clean the hair, then condition the hair in the rinse phase also are good choices.

- Look for products containing dimethicone, which is available in shampoos, conditioners, sprays, and creams. This ingredient has been shown to decrease static electricity, increase shine, and improve manageability.

- Try newly introduced hair serums, which are applied by a few drops on the hands and rubbed through the length of the hair (but should not be applied directly to the scalp).

- Stop dyeing your hair and opt for hair's natural hair color instead.

- If you must dye your hair, stay "on shade"—or dye the hair within three color shades of its natural color. Dyeing hair darker, rather than lighter, also is generally better.

When The Heat Is On, Hair Needs Some Time Off

Heat damage is another common source of hair damage, which produces a condition known as bubble hair. This occurs when the water in the hair, which makes the hair flexible, gets heated and turns into steam. Hair bubbles then occur on the hair shaft, creating a loss of cuticle. Signs of this form of hair damage include hair that smells burned, frizzy ends, and hair that breaks easily.

"Dramatic temperature changes are hard on hair, and heat can, in a sense, cook the hair," said Dr. Draelos. "Think of hair like a piece of steak—it starts out nice and soft and flexible. But when you cook it, the steak changes texture and becomes hard. Similarly, hair transforms when exposed to heat over time, resulting in brittle hair that breaks easily. Protecting hair from too much heat is essential to maintaining healthy hair."

Hair damaged by heat cannot be repaired, as the affected hair will need to be cut off and allowed to regrow as healthy hair. Allow hair to air dry, when possible.

Dr. Draelos offered these tips for heat-damaged hair:

- Allow hair to air dry when possible.

- When using a hairdryer, do not use the highest heat setting immediately. Start out on the lowest heat setting first, then gradually increase heat.

- To straighten hair with a ceramic iron, put a moist towel in the device to protect the hair from direct heat.

- Look for temperature-controlled devices to control the amount of direct heat to hair.

- Moisturizing the hair regularly will help the appearance of heat-damaged hair to some degree, but stopping the source of heat damage is essential.

Straightening Hair Comes At A Price

While ceramic flat irons are quite popular with women seeking sleek, straight hair, another procedure that uses chemicals in combination with heat to straighten or rearrange the hair's natural bonds is known as keratin hair straightening. Typically performed in salons, keratin hair straightening uses glutaraldehyde or formaldehyde rather than lye—a stronger bond breaker also used for hair straightening but which is even more damaging—combed through the hair to make it straight.

After one of the chemical solutions is applied to the hair, a keratin protein conditioner is put on the hair to make it less brittle. With this procedure, hair must be kept dry and not bent or manipulated for several days after the process.

For women considering keratin hair straightening, Dr. Draelos offered these suggestions:

- Avoid this procedure if you have tightly kinked hair, as it will not work in rearranging the natural hair bonds.

- To minimize hair damage and loss, extend the time between treatments.

- When washing hair, use a generous amount of conditioner to make hair less brittle.

- If hair becomes frizzy and brittle, stop the procedure and let new hair growth replace damaged hair.

TLC For Healthy Hair

To keep healthy hair looking its best, Dr. Draelos also provided the following tips:

- The less you do to your hair, the better. Avoid over-styling or processing hair.

- Be sure to wash the scalp, which is where the oil is, and then let shampoo run through the hair. Shampoo is meant to clean the scalp primarily and can damage the hair if overused.

- Let how oily your scalp is determine how often you wash your hair. If your scalp is oily, wash hair more frequently than if the scalp was drier.

- Conditioner should be used on the ends of the hair, not on the scalp, for best results.

- Pick a shampoo and conditioner based on your hair shape, such as curly or straight, and your hair condition, such as damaged, fine, or frizzy. These products don't need to be expensive to work well for your hair.

- Wear a hat to protect hair from ultraviolet (UV) radiation.

"It is best to choose a hairstyle closest to your hair's natural structure and color as possible, which will minimize hair damage," added Dr. Draelos. "Be sure to consult your dermatologist for any questions about styling products, concerns about the appearance of your hair, or unexplained hair loss."

Chapter 62

Unwanted Hair: Removing Hair Safely

The U.S. Food and Drug Administration's (FDA) Center for Devices and Radiological Health regulates electrolysis equipment and lasers. Chemical depilatories, waxes, and shaving creams and gels fall under the jurisdiction of FDA's Office of Cosmetics and Colors in the Center for Food Safety and Applied Nutrition. The practice of professional hair removal is generally regulated by state and local authorities. Here are some tips related to common methods of hair removal.

Laser Hair Removal

In this method, a laser destroys hair follicles with heat.

Sometimes it is recommended that a topical anesthetic product be used before a laser hair removal procedure, to minimize pain. In these cases, FDA recommends that consumers discuss with a medical professional the circumstances under which the cream should be used, and whether the use is appropriate.

Those who decide to use a skin-numbing product should follow the directions of a healthcare provider and consider using a product that contains the lowest amount of anesthetic drugs possible. FDA's Center for Drug Evaluation and Research has received reports of serious and life-threatening side effects after use of large amounts of skin-numbing products for laser hair removal.

Side effects of laser hair removal can include blistering, discoloration after treatment, swelling, redness, and scarring. Sunlight should be avoided during healing after the procedure.

About This Chapter: Excerpted from "Removing Hair Safely," Center for Devices and Radiological Health, CFSAN/Office of Cosmetics and Color, U.S. Food and Drug Administration (www.fda.gov), August 9, 2012.

Epilators: Needle, Electrolysis, And Tweezers

Needle epilators introduce a fine wire close to the hair shaft, under the skin, and into the hair follicle. An electric current travels down the wire and destroys the hair root at the bottom of the follicle, and the loosened hair is removed with tweezers.

Medical electrolysis devices destroy hair growth with a shortwave radio frequency after a thin probe is placed in the hair follicle. Risks from these methods include infection from an unsterile needle and scarring from improper technique. Electrolysis is considered a permanent hair removal method, since it destroys the hair follicle. It requires a series of appointments over a period of time.

Tweezer epilators also use electric current to remove hair. The tweezers grasp the hair close to the skin, and energy is applied at the tip of the tweezer. There is no body of significant information establishing the effectiveness of the tweezer epilator to permanently remove hair.

Depilatories

Available in gel, cream, lotion, aerosol, and roll-on forms, depilatories are highly alkaline (or, in some cases, acidic) formulations that affect the protein structure of the hair, causing it to dissolve into a jellylike mass that the user can easily wipe from the skin. Consumers should carefully follow instructions and heed all warnings on the product label.

For example, manufacturers typically recommend conducting a preliminary skin test for allergic reaction and irritation. Depilatories should not be used for eyebrows or around eyes or on inflamed or broken skin.

FDA's Office of Cosmetics and Colors has received reports of burns, blisters, stinging, itchy rashes, and skin peeling associated with depilatories and other types of cosmetic hair removers.

Waxing, Sugaring, And Threading

Unlike chemical depilatories that remove hair at the skin's surface, these methods pluck hairs out of the follicle, below the surface.

With waxing, a layer of melted wax is applied to the skin and allowed to harden. (Cold waxes, which are soft at room temperature, allow the user to skip the steps of melting and hardening.) It is then pulled off quickly in the opposite direction of the hair growth, taking the uprooted hair with it. Labeling of waxes may caution that these products should not be used by people with diabetes and circulatory problems. Waxes should not be used over varicose veins, moles, or warts. Waxes also shouldn't be used on eyelashes, the nose, ears, or on nipples, genital areas, or on irritated, chapped, or sunburned skin. As with chemical depilatories, it can be a good idea to do a preliminary test on a small area for allergic reaction or irritation.

Sugaring is similar to waxing. A heated sugar mixture is spread on the skin, sometimes covered with a strip of fabric, and then lifted off to remove hair. Threading is an ancient technique in which a loop of thread is rotated across the skin to pluck the hair. All of these techniques may cause skin irritation and infection.

Shaving

Shaving hair only when it's wet, and shaving in the direction in which the hairs lie, can help lessen skin irritation and cuts. It's important to use a clean razor with a sharp blade. Contrary to popular belief, shaving does not change the texture, color, or growth rate of hair. Razors and electric shavers are under the jurisdiction of the Consumer Product Safety Commission.

Chapter 63

Your Feet Need Care, Too

Summer Feet Tips

Use these 10 summer foot care tips from The Society of Chiropodists & Podiatrists to get your feet in shape for summer.

1. Trim Your Toenails For Summer

Use proper nail clippers and cut straight across, not too short, and not down at the corners as this can lead to ingrown nails. File them, if that's easier.

2. Go Barefoot

Go barefoot or wear open-toed sandals whenever you can in the hot weather (except when you're in a communal shower or changing area) to help stop your feet getting sweaty and smelly.

3. Forget Flip-Flops

Don't be tempted to wear flip-flops all through the summer. They don't provide support for your feet and can give you arch and heel pain if you wear them for too long.

4. Change Socks Daily

If you have to wear socks in hot weather, change them once a day and choose ones that contain at least 70 percent cotton or wool to keep your feet dry and stop them from smelling.

About This Chapter: This chapter begins with "Summer Feet Tips," reprinted from NHS Choices, www.nhs.uk. Reproduced by kind permission of the Department of Health, © 2013.

5. Remove Hard Skin

Hard, cracked skin around the heels is very common in summer, often caused by open-backed sandals and flip-flops rubbing around the edge of the heel. Use a foot file, emery board, or pumice stone to gently rub away the hard skin, then apply a rich moisturizing cream such as aqueous cream or E45 to soften the skin.

6. Banish Blisters

Blisters strike more often in hot weather. They're caused by rubbing, especially between the toes if you're wearing flip-flops with "thongs." Lorraine Jones, a podiatrist from The Society of Chiropodists & Podiatrists, says the key to preventing summer blisters is to keep your feet dry, wear shoes or sandals that fit well and aren't too loose, and give your feet ample rest so they don't get hot and sweaty. If you do get a blister, don't put a bandage over it. Leave it to dry out on its own.

7. Ring The Changes

Wear a variety of different sandals and shoes during summer to help prevent cracked heels, hard skin and blisters. Lorraine says: "We understand that when the summer arrives, people are naturally going to opt for lightweight footwear such as flip-flops and flimsy sandals. However, we'd recommend alternating your footwear so that you aren't wearing this style of shoe day in and day out."

8. Watch Out For Foot Infections

The floors of communal showers and changing rooms at open-air and hotel swimming pools are hot spots for infections such as athlete's foot and verrucas. Don't wander around public pools barefoot. Protect your feet by wearing flip-flops in the changing room and at the pool edge.

9. Tackle Sweat

If you have sweaty feet in the summer, it's even more important to wash your feet each morning and evening in warm, soapy water then dry them thoroughly. You can also use an antibacterial wash, which helps deal with foot odor. Then wipe them with cotton wool dipped in surgical spirit and dust them with talc.

10. Get Help If You Need It

Basic hygiene and nail cutting should be all you need to keep your feet healthy. But if you have any problems, such as hard skin that you can't get rid of, it's best to seek professional help.

Your GP (family doctor) will be able to advise you on local foot services.

Registered podiatrists (also known as chiropodists) are trained in all aspects of care for the feet. The Society of Chiropodists & Podiatrists (based in the United Kingdom) can help you find a local podiatrist.

You may be able to get NHS (based in the United Kingdom) treatment from a podiatrist or chiropodist. Some NHS podiatry services offer self-referral, so you don't have to go through your GP.

Foot Care And Diabetes

Source: Text under this heading is excerpted from "Prevent Diabetes Problems: Keep Your Feet And Skin Healthy," National Institute of Diabetes and Digestive and Kidney Diseases (www.niddk.nih.gov), May 2008. Reviewed by David A. Cooke, MD, FACP, February 25, 2013.

How can diabetes hurt my feet?

High blood glucose from diabetes causes two problems that can hurt your feet:

- **Nerve Damage:** One problem is damage to nerves in your legs and feet. With damaged nerves, you might not feel pain, heat, or cold in your legs and feet. A sore or cut on your foot may get worse because you do not know it is there. This lack of feeling is caused by nerve damage, also called diabetic neuropathy. Nerve damage can lead to a sore or an infection.

- **Poor Blood Flow:** The second problem happens when not enough blood flows to your legs and feet. Poor blood flow makes it hard for a sore or infection to heal.

Skin-Care Tips For People With Diabetes

- After you wash with a mild soap, make sure you rinse and dry yourself well. Check places where water can hide, such as under the arms, under the breasts, between the legs, and between the toes.

- Keep your skin moist by using a lotion or cream after you wash. Ask your doctor to suggest one.

- Drink lots of fluids, such as water, to keep your skin moist and healthy.

- Check your skin after you wash. Make sure you have no dry, red, or sore spots that might lead to an infection.

- Tell your doctor about any skin problems.

Source: Excerpted from "Prevent Diabetes Problems: Keep Your Feet And Skin Healthy," National Institute of Diabetes and Digestive and Kidney Diseases (www.niddk.nih.gov), May 2008. Reviewed by David A. Cooke, MD, FACP, February 25, 2013.

What can I do to take care of my feet?

- **Wash your feet in warm water every day.** Make sure the water is not too hot by testing the temperature with your elbow. Do not soak your feet. Dry your feet well, especially between your toes.

- **Look at your feet every day to check for cuts, sores, blisters, redness, calluses, or other problems.** Checking every day is even more important if you have nerve damage or poor blood flow.

- **If your skin is dry, rub lotion on your feet after you wash and dry them.** Do not put lotion between your toes.

- **File corns and calluses gently with an emery board or pumice stone.** Do this after your bath or shower.

- **Cut your toenails once a week or when needed.** Cut toenails when they are soft from washing. Cut them to the shape of the toe and not too short. File the edges with an emery board.

- **Always wear slippers or shoes to protect your feet from injuries.**

- **Always wear socks or stockings to avoid blisters.** Do not wear socks or knee-high stockings that are too tight below your knee.

- **Wear shoes that fit well.** Shop for shoes at the end of the day when your feet are bigger. Break in shoes slowly. Wear them one to two hours each day for the first few weeks.

- **Before putting your shoes on, feel the insides to make sure they have no sharp edges or objects that might injure your feet.**

What are common diabetes foot problems?

Anyone can have corns, blisters, and other foot problems. If you have diabetes and your blood glucose stays high, these foot problems can lead to infections. See Figures 63.1–5 for more information about common foot problems.

How can my doctor help me take care of my feet?

- Tell your doctor right away about any foot problems.

- Your doctor should do a complete foot exam every year.

- Ask your doctor to look at your feet at each diabetes checkup. To make sure your doctor checks your feet, take off your shoes and socks before your doctor comes into the room.

Figure 63.1. Corns and calluses are thick layers of skin caused by too much rubbing or pressure on the same spot. Corns and calluses can become infected.

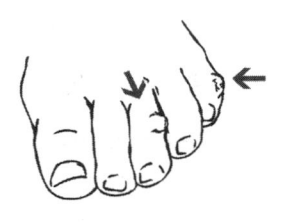

Figure 63.2. Blisters can form if shoes always rub the same spot. Wearing shoes that do not fit or wearing shoes without socks can cause blisters. Blisters can become infected.

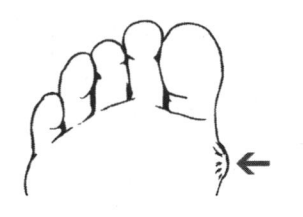

Figure 63.3. Ingrown toenails happen when an edge of the nail grows into the skin. The skin can get red and infected. Ingrown toenails can happen if you cut into the corners of your toenails when you trim them. You can also get an ingrown toenail if your shoes are too tight. If toenail edges are sharp, smooth them with an emery board.

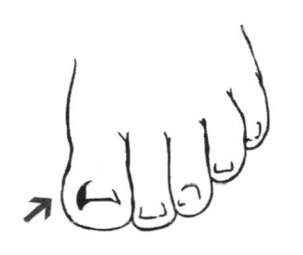

Figure 63.4. A bunion forms when your big toe slants toward the small toes and the place between the bones near the base of your big toe grows big. This spot can get red, sore, and infected. Bunions can form on one or both feet. Pointed shoes may cause bunions. Bunions often run in the family. Surgery can remove bunions.

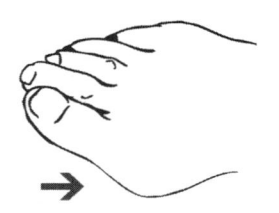

Figure.63.5 Plantar warts are caused by a virus. The warts usually form on the bottoms of the feet.

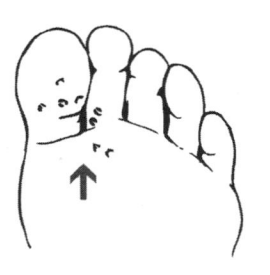

Source for Figures 63.1–5: National Institute of Diabetes and Digestive and Kidney Diseases, May 2008. Reviewed by David A. Cooke, MD, FACP, February 25, 2013.

- Ask your doctor to check how well the nerves in your feet sense feeling.

- Ask your doctor to check how well blood is flowing to your legs and feet.

- Ask your doctor to show you the best way to trim your toenails. Ask what lotion or cream to use on your legs and feet.

- If you cannot cut your toenails or you have a foot problem, ask your doctor to send you to a foot doctor. A doctor who cares for feet is called a podiatrist.

How can special shoes help my feet?

Special shoes can be made to fit softly around your sore feet or feet that have changed shape. These special shoes help protect your feet. Medicare and other health insurance programs may pay for special shoes. Talk with your doctor about how and where to get them.

Chapter 64

Nail Care And Health

Nails are a specialized form of skin. They provide 10 (or 20) little places that you can decorate. But more than that, they protect your sensitive fingers and toes, and they help you pick up small things, scratch itches, and hold on to or manipulate objects. You can also abuse them by biting, peeling, and picking at them.

Nail Care And Grooming

Your nails provide important clues to your overall health. Broken, discolored, or misshapen nails can indicate nutritional deficiencies, infections, or skin conditions. Good nail care keeps your hands and feet looking nice and is part of a general program of good health habits.

Basic tips to care for your nails include the following:

- Keep them clean and dry. This helps prevent infection.

- Shape them straight across rather than to a point. Pointed nails are weaker and can break more easily.

- Do not bite or pick them. Bitten nails are more easily infected.

Nail Polish And Removers

Nail polishes and removers are chemical lacquers, hardeners and solvents. U.S Food and Drug Administration (FDA)-approved nail products are safe to use, but some people have allergic reactions to some of the chemicals.

About This Chapter: From "Caring For Nails For Teenagers: Grooming, Manicures, And Problems," reprinted with permission from the Palo Alto Medical Foundation Teen Health website, http://www.pamf.org/teen. © 2012 Palo Alto Medical Foundation. All rights reserved.

Acetone, a common solvent in nail polish remover, can dry your nails, making them brittle and prone to splitting and breaking. Also, one compound used in some acrylic nails, methacrylate (MMA), has caused allergic reactions so severe that people have lost entire nails, causing it to be banned in many states. Check with your local salon stores before allowing them to do work on your nails. If your nail salon does use MMA, ask them if they have an alternative product. It's not worth risking the loss of your nails!

Artificial Nails And Manicures

Artificial nails and manicures are very popular and can help your hands look nice. However, they can also be a source of health problems.

Manicure tools and instruments used in salons are used on many different people. If these tools are not properly sterilized, you can get an infection including: HIV, hepatitis B or C, or warts.

If you have your nails professionally applied or manicured, you should check to make sure the manicurists sterilize their equipment after each use. An alternative would be to take your own manicure tools for the manicurist to use.

Nail Problems

Because they're right out there on the ends of our hands and feet, nails are subject to a lot of abuse. Some of the abuse, like biting, is self-inflicted. But everyone has experienced broken or ripped nails from catching them on or in something, or cracking and splitting from overexposure to water and chemicals.

Minor nail problems usually heal as the nail grows out and require little treatment other than perhaps protecting the finger or toe if it is especially sensitive. In addition to allergic reactions to nail cosmetics and chemicals, there are a few other common problems that can occur with nails.

- **Abuse—Biting, Picking, And Peeling:** When you bite your nails, you are interfering with their ability to protect your sensitive fingers. What's more, you are inviting infection. Your nails can become infected because the surface is either broken or removed. You can also be eating all kinds of nasty things that may be under your nails from things you have touched during the day. If you touch your dog, your car, or your schoolbooks, and then bite your nails, you are ingesting the same kinds of things you would if you had licked these objects. Pretty disgusting, huh? In addition, bitten-down nails are not very attractive.

- **Fungal Infections:** A fungal infection occurs when a fungus attacks a fingernail, a toenail, or the skin under the nail. You can get fungal infections from walking barefoot in public showers or pools. If you have athlete's foot, the fungus can spread from your skin to your nails.

- **Color Changes:** Nails may sometimes change in color as a result of an injury, some medications, nutritional imbalances, or skin conditions. If the color of your nails has changed dramatically, it is a good idea to check with your doctor.

- **Hangnails:** The skin around your nails can become irritated and infected from biting or chewing, minor injuries, or exposure to water and chemicals. Hangnails can cause soreness around your nails, and if an infection develops you should see your doctor.

- **Ingrown Nails:** These can be painful. They are usually caused by improper trimming of the nail or by wearing shoes that are too tight. If you have an ingrown toenail, do not attempt to treat it yourself by cutting or digging at it. Have it treated properly by your doctor.

Part Seven
If You Need More Information

Chapter 65

Additional Reading About Skin Concerns

Acne And Rosacea

Nodulocystic Acne. New Zealand Dermatological Society. As of February 25, 2013: http://www
.dermnetnz.org/acne/nodulocystic-acne.html

Rosacea: Your Self-Help Guide. Brownstein, Arlen, and Donna Shoemaker. Oakland, CA: New
Harbinger Publications, 2001.

Ethnicity And Skin

Treating Acne in Skin of Color. American Academy of Dermatology. As of February 25, 2013:
http://www.skincarephysicians.com/acnenet/article_skinofcolor.html

Dr. Susan Taylor's Rx for Brown Skin: Your Prescription for Flawless Skin, Hair, and Nails. Taylor,
Susan C. New York, NY: Amistad, 2008.

Hair And Nail Care

Hair Care on a Budget. American Academy of Dermatology. As of February 25, 2013: http://
www.aad.org/stories-and-news/news-releases/hair-care-on-a-budget.

Nails. American Academy of Dermatology. As of February 25, 2013: http://www.aad.org/media
-resources/stats-and-facts/prevention-and-care/nails/nails

Hair Loss

Alopecia Areata: Understanding and Coping with Hair Loss. Thompson, Wendy, and Jerry Shapiro. Baltimore, MD: Johns Hopkins University Press, 1996.

Frequently Asked Questions. National Alopecia Areata Foundation. As of February 25, 2013: http://www.naaf.org/site/PageServer?pagename=about_alopecia_faq

Lupus

Living With Lupus: The Complete Guide, 2nd ed. Blau, Sheldon Paul, and Dodi Schultz. Cambridge, MA, 2004.

The Lupus Book: A Guide for Patients and Their Families. Wallace, Daniel J. New York, NY: Oxford University Press, 2012.

Skin Cancer

100 Questions & Answers about Melanoma and Other Skin Cancers. McClay, Edward F., Mary-Ellen T. McClay, and Jodie Smith. Sudbury, MA: Jones and Bartlett Publishers, 2004.

Actinic Keratosis (AK). Skin Cancer Foundation. As of February 25, 2013: http://www.skin cancer.org/skin-cancer-information/actinic-keratosis

Early Detection and Self Exams. Skin Cancer Foundation. As of February 25, 2013: http://www .skincancer.org/skin-cancer-information/early-detection

Saving Your Skin: Prevention, Early Detection, and Treatment of Melanoma and Other Skin Cancers. Kenet, Barney, and Patricia Lawler. New York, NY: Four Walls Eight Windows, 1998.

Skin Cancer. National Cancer Institute. As of February 25, 2013: http://www.cancer.gov/cancer topics/types/skin

Skin Cancer: Prevention Guidelines. Skin Cancer Foundation. As of February 25, 2013: http:// www.skincancer.org/prevention/sun-protection/prevention-guidelines

How to Perform a Self-Exam (Video). American Academy of Dermatology. As of February 25, 2013: http://www.aad.org/spot-skin-cancer/understanding-skin-cancer/how-do-i-check-my -skin/how-to-perform-a-self-exam

Sunbeds. World Health Organization. As of February 25, 2013: http://www.who.int/uv/faq/ sunbeds/en/index5.html

Understanding Basal Cell Carcinoma: What You Need to Know. Robbins, Perry. New York, NY: Skin Cancer Foundation, 2006.

Understanding Skin Cancer. American Academy of Dermatology. As of February 25, 2013: http://www.aad.org/spot-skin-cancer/understanding-skin-cancer

Understanding Squamous Cell Carcinoma: What You Need to Know. Robbins, Perry. New York, NY: Skin Cancer Foundation, 2006.

Skin Care And Cosmetic Procedures

Body Art Fact Sheet: Took Kit for Teen Care, Second Edition. American College of Obstetricians and Gynecologists. As of February 25, 2013: http://www.acog.org/~/media/Departments/Adolescent%20Health%20Care/Teen%20Care%20Tool%20Kit/BodyArt.pdf?dmc=1&ts=20130225T1333597281

A Consumer's Dictionary of Cosmetic Ingredients, 7th Edition: Complete Information About the Harmful and Desirable Ingredients Found in Cosmetics and Cosmeceuticals. Winter, Ruth. New York, NY: Three Rivers Press, 2009.

Don't Go to the Cosmetics Counter Without Me, 9th ed. Begoun, Paula, Bryan Barton, and Desiree Stordahl. Renton, WA: Beginning Press, 2012.

Encyclopedia of Body Adornment. DeMello, Margo. Westport, CT: Greenwood Press, 2007.

The Original Beauty Bible: Skin Care Facts for Ageless Beauty, 3rd ed. Begoun, Paula. Seattle, WA: Beginning Press, 2009.

The Piercing Bible: The Definitive Guide to Safe Body Piercing. Angel, Elayne. Berkeley, CA: Crossing Press, 2013.

A Practical Guide to Chemical Peels, Microdermabrasion & Topical Products. Small, Rebecca. Philadelphia, PA: Lippincott, 2012.

The Skin Type Solution. Baumann, Leslie. New York, NY: Bantam Books, 2006.

Teens and Plastic Surgery. American Society for Aesthetic Plastic Surgery. As of February 25, 2013: http://www.surgery.org/media/news-releases/teens-and-plastic-surgery

Skin—Psychological Issues

Psychodermatology: The Psychological Impact of Skin Disorders. Edited by Walker, Carl, and Linda Papadopoulos. New York, NY: Cambridge University Press, 2005.

Trichotillomania, Skin Picking, and Other Body-Focused Repetitive Behavior. Grant, Jon E., Dan J. Stein, Douglas W. Woods, and Nancy J. Keuthen. Arlington, VA: American Psychiatric Publishing, 2011.

Skin—Related Diseases And Problems

Living With Skin Conditions (Teen's Guides). Chamlin, Sarah L., and E.A. Tremblay. New York, NY: Checkmark Books, 2010.

The Lyme Disease Solution. Singleton, Kenneth B. Charleston, SC: BookSurge Publishing, 2008.

Questions & Answers About Human Papilloma Virus (HPV). Dizon, Don S., and Michael L. Krychman. Sudbury, MA: Jones and Bartlett Publishers, 2011.

Psoriasis: Everything You Need to Know. Langley, Richard. Buffalo, NY: Firefly Books, 2005.

The Scleroderma Book: A Guide for Patients and Families. Mayes, Maureen. New York, NY: Oxford University Press, 2005.

Severe Burns: A Family Guide to Medical and Emotional Recovery. Munster, Andrew M., and Baltimore Regional Burn Center Staff. Baltimore, MD: Johns Hopkins University Press, 1993.

Skin Disease and Skin Condition List. Skinsight. As of February 25, 2013: Click on "Disease Name" in left column for illustrations and text on specific conditions. http://www.skinsight.com/diseaseList.htm

Skin—General Information

Andrews' Diseases of the Skin: Clinical Dermatology—Expert Consult, 11th ed. James, William D., Timothy G. Berger, and Dirk M. Elston. Philadelphia, PA: Saunders Elsevier, 2011.

Fitzpatrick's Color Atlas and Synopsis of Clinical Dermatology, 7th ed. Wolff, Klaus, and Richard A. Johnson. New York, NY: McGraw Hill, 2013.

The Skin You're In: Teaching Guide for Preteens and Young Teens. American Skin Association. As of February 25, 2013: http://www.americanskin.org/education/the_skin_youre_in/pdf/teaching_guide.pdf

Teenage Skin. American Academy of Dermatology. As of February 25, 2013: http://www.aad.org/media-resources/stats-and-facts/prevention-and-care/teenage-skin

Chapter 66

Resources For Skin Information

American Academy of Dermatology

P.O. Box 4014
Schaumburg, IL 60168
Toll-Free: 866-503-SKIN (866-503-7546)
Phone: 847-240-1280
Fax: 847-240-1859
Website: http://www.aad.org
E-mail: mrc@aad.org

American Academy of Facial Plastic and Reconstructive Surgery

310 South Henry Street
Alexandria, VA 22314
Phone: 703-299-9291
Fax: 703-299-8898
Website: http://www.aafprs.org
E-mail: info@aafprs.org

American Academy of Family Physicians

11400 Tomahawk Creek Parkway
Leawood, KS 66211-2680
Toll-Free: 800-274-2237
Phone: 913-906-6000
Fax: 913-906-6075
Website: http://www.aafp.org

American Academy of Pediatrics

141 Northwest Point Boulevard
Elk Grove Village, IL 60007-1098
Phone: 847-434-4000
Fax: 847-434-8000
Website: http://www.healthychildren.org
E-mail: info@healthychildren.org

About This Chapter: Resources in this chapter were compiled from multiple sources deemed reliable. Inclusion does not constitute endorsement, and there is no implication associated with omission. All contact information was verified and updated in February 2013.

American Lyme Disease Foundation

P.O. Box 466
Lyme, CT 06371
Website: http://www.aldf.com
E-mail: questions@aldf.com

American Osteopathic College of Dermatology

1501 East Illinois Street
P.O. Box 7525
Kirksville, MO 63501
Toll-Free: 800-449-2623
Phone: 660-665-2184
Fax: 660-627-2623
Website: http://www.aocd.org
E-mail: info@aocd.org

American Skin Association

6 East 43rd Street, 28th Floor
New York, NY 10017
Toll-Free: 800-499-SKIN
(800-499-7546)
Phone: 212-889-4858
Fax: 212-889-4959
Website: http://www.americanskin.org
E-mail: info@americanskin.org

American Society for Dermatological Surgery

5550 Meadowbrook Drive, Suite 120
Rolling Meadows, IL 60008
Phone: 847-956-0900
Fax: 847-956-0999
Website: http://www.asds.net

American Society of Plastic Surgeons

444 East Algonquin Road
Arlington Heights, IL 60005
Phone: 847-228-9900
Website: http://www.plasticsurgery.org

Asthma and Allergy Foundation of America

8201 Corporate Drive, Suite 1000
Landover, MD 20785
Toll-Free: 800-7-ASTHMA
(800-727-8462)
Website: http://www.aafa.org
E-mail: Info@aafa.org

Center for Young Women's Health

333 Longwood Avenue, 5th Floor
Boston, MA 02115
Phone: 617-355-2994
Fax: 617-730-0186
Website: http://www.
youngwomenshealth.org

Centers for Disease Control and Prevention (CDC)

1600 Clifton Road
Atlanta, GA 30333
Toll-Free: 800-CDC-INFO
(800-232-4636)
Toll-Free TTY: 888-232-6348
Website: http://www.cdc.gov
E-mail: cdcinfo@cdc.gov

Cleveland Clinic Foundation

9500 Euclid Avenue
Cleveland, OH 44195
Phone: 216-444-2200
Toll-Free: 800-223-2273
TTY: 216-444-0261
Website: http://www.clevelandclinic.org

Federal Trade Commission (FTC)

600 Pennsylvania Avenue NW
Washington, DC 20580
Phone: 202-326-2222
Website: http://www.ftc.gov

Food and Drug Administration (FDA)

10903 New Hampshire Avenue
Silver Spring, MD 20993
Toll-Free: 888-INFO-FDA
(888-463-6332)
Website: http://www.fda.gov

Hampton University Skin of Color Research Institute

P.O. Box 6035
Hampton, VA 23668
Phone: 757-727-5885
Website: http://huscri.org
E-mail: info@huscri.org

International Hyperhidrosis Society

2560 Township Road, Suite B
Quakertown, PA 18951
Phone: 610-346-6008
Website: http://www.sweathelp.org
Email: info@sweathelp.org

Louisiana State University School of Veterinary Medicine

Skip Bertman Drive
Baton Rouge, LA 70803
Phone: 225-578-9900
Fax: 225-578-9916
Website: http://www.vetmed.lsu.edu
E-mail: svmweb@vetmed.lsu.edu

Lupus Foundation of America

2000 L Street NW, Suite 410
Washington, DC 20036
Toll-Free: 800-558-0121
Phone: 202-349-1155
Fax: 202-349-1156
Website: http://www.lupus.org
E-mail: info@lupus

National Alopecia Areata Foundation

14 Mitchell Boulevard
San Rafael, CA 94903
Phone: 415-472-3780
Fax: 415-472-5343
Website: http://www.naaf.org
E-mail: info@naaf.org

National Cancer Institute

6116 Executive Boulevard
Suite 300
Bethesda, MD 20892-832214
Toll-Free: 800-4-CANCER
(800-422-6237)
Website: http://www.cancer.gov

National Eczema Association

4460 Redwood Highway
Suite 16D
San Rafael, CA 94903-1953
Toll-Free: 800-818-7546
Phone: 415-499-3474
Website: http://www.nationaleczema.org
E-mail: info@nationaleczema.org

National Institute of Allergy and Infectious Diseases (NIAID)

6610 Rockledge Drive
MSC 6612
Bethesda, MD 20892-6612
Toll-Free: 866-284-4107
Toll-Free TDD: 800-877-8339
Phone: 301-496-5717
Fax: 301-402-3573
Website: http://www.niaid.nih.gov
E-mail: ocpostoffice@niaid.nih.gov

National Institute of Arthritis and Musculoskeletal and Skin Diseases (NIAMS)

1 AMS Circle
Bethesda, MD 20892-3675
Toll-Free: 877-22-NIAMS
(877-226-4267)
Phone: 301-495-4484
TTY: 301-565-2966
Fax: 301-718-6366
Website: http://www.niams.nih.gov
E-mail: NIAMSinfo@mail.nih.gov

National Library of Medicine

Reference and Web Services
8600 Rockville Pike
Bethesda, MD 20894
Toll-Free: 888-FIND-NLM
(888-346-3656)
Toll-Free TDD: 800-735-2258
(via Maryland Relay Service)
Phone: 301-594-5983
Fax: 301-402-1384
Website: http://www.nlm.nih.gov
E-mail: custserv@nlm.nih.gov

National Psoriasis Foundation

6600 SW 92nd Avenue, Suite 300
Portland, OR 97223
Toll-Free: 800-723-9166
Phone: 503-244-7404
Fax: 503-245-0626
Website: http://www.psoriasis.org
E-mail: getinfo@psoriasis.org

National Rosacea Society
196 James Street
Barrington, IL 60010
Toll-Free: 888-NO-BLUSH
(888-662-5874)
Fax: 847-382-5567
Website: http://www.rosacea.org
E-mail: rosaceas@aol.com

Nemours Foundation
10140 Centurion Parkway
Jacksonville, FL 32256
Phone: 904-697-4100
Website: http://www.nemours.org

New Zealand Dermatological Society
P.O. Box 4431
Palmerston North
New Zealand
Phone: 06 357-1466
Fax: 06 357-1426
Website: http://www.dermnetnz.org

Office on Women's Health
U.S. Department of Health and Human Services
200 Independence Avenue SW
Room 712E
Washington, DC 20201
Toll-Free: 800-994-9662
Phone: 202-690-7650
Fax: 202-205-2631
Website: http://www.womenshealth.gov

Scleroderma Foundation
300 Rosewood Drive
Suite 105
Danvers, MA 01923
Toll-Free: 800-722-HOPE
(800-722-4673)
Phone: 978-463-5843
Fax: 978-463-5809
Website: http://www.scleroderma.org
E-mail: sfinfo@scleroderma.org

Skin Cancer Foundation
149 Madison Avenue
Suite 901
New York, NY 10016
Phone: 212-725-5176
Website: http://www.skincancer.org

Trichotillomania Learning Center (TLC)
207 McPherson Street
Suite H
Santa Cruz, CA 95060-5863
Phone: 831-457-1004
Fax: 831-427-5541 fax
Website: http://www.trich.org
E-mail: info@trich.org

Vitiligo Support International
P.O. Box 3565
Lynchburg, VA 24503
Phone: 434-326-5380
Website: http://www.vitiligosupport.org

Women's Dermatologic Society (WDS)

700 North Fairfax Street
Suite 510
Alexandria, VA 22314
Toll-Free: 877-WDS-ROSE
(877-937-7673)
Phone: 571-527-3115
Fax: 571-527-3105
Website: http://www.womensderm.org
E-mail: wds@womensderm.org

Index

Index

Page numbers that appear in *Italics* refer to tables or illustrations. Page numbers that have a small 'n' after the page number refer to citation information shown as Notes. Page numbers that appear in **Bold** refer to information contained in boxes on that page (except Notes information at the beginning of each chapter).

A

C